What others are saying about this book:

"A unique and helpful guide to timeless, classic style."
> — **Dr. Judith A. Schwartz, Executive Director,
> Lifelong Learning Institute at
> Washington University in St. Louis**

"With Corinne Richardson's hands-on approach to creating a simple wardrobe, you'll be comfortably and stylishly dressed for every occasion."
> — **Fran Santoro Hamilton, author of *Hands-On English***

"At last, a simple, easy, and sophisticated way to dress so we can relax and continue to carry on with our lives in style!"
> — **Marcella E. Widdoes, Editor of *A Sampler
> From Marcy's*, a bi-lingual presentation
> of international cuisine**

"Tired of the same old advice about clothes? Read this book for fresh, new ideas."
> — **Debra Van Elslander, former assistant to the
> Chairman of Art Van Furniture Company of
> Warren, Michigan for 25 years**

"An elegant way to simplify your life is to simplify your wardrobe."
> — **Dr. Karen Goodhope, radiologist**

"With *Dressing Nifty*, you learn the secrets to smart shopping and effortless dressing."

**— Adrienne Fairbanks, RN,
President of Asure Test, Inc.**

"A book that delivers simplicity, style, and self-assurance in choosing a wardrobe is a treasure. The advice in *Dressing Nifty After Fifty* is universal, yet tailor-made for each reader."

— Bobbi Linkemer, author of *How to Write a Nonfiction Book From Concept to Completion in 6 months*

"Keeping our wardrobes on track is a challenge for working women. This book shows us how."

**— Sue Harrison, Loan Closing Manager,
GE Real Estate**

"This book tells all about dressing with simple elegance, taste, and ease."

**— Nancy A. Sachar, former Chief Deputy Clerk,
Missouri Court of Appeals, Eastern District**

"With graceful, concise language, Corinne Richardson not only details the steps to assemble a flattering wardrobe, but also engages the reader's imagination in the process. The result is not only a more attractive look but also a greater sense of individuality for the wearer."

**— Sandy Van Arsdale, Dielmann Sotheby's
International Realty**

"Corinne Richardson takes the mystery out of building and maintaining a wardrobe."

— Linda Wheatley, psychologist, teacher, author

"Terrific book — packed with helpful ideas."

— Marie Dargan, former Director of Delinquency Services, St. Louis County Family Court

"By learning how to be in style from this well-written book, I and other readers will look better and feel better about ourselves!"

— Ellen Brasunas, Licensed Professional Counselor

"Corinne Richardson understands the fine art of a sophisticated, uncomplicated wardrobe."

— Louise T. Hall, ASA, appraiser of antiques & decorative arts

"Corinne Richardson has created an invaluable guide for women committed to living their lives in an intentional manner. Her recommendations are straightforward and can make the critical difference in the quality of how we present ourselves to both ourselves and to the world at large."

— Andrea Bull, former Director of Human Resources, Barnes Jewish Hospital, St. Louis, MO, and Current Owner, AB Senior Services, LLC

"How nice to laugh as I consider the different ways to stay in style."

— Rita Fineberg, accountant

DRESSING NIFTY AFTER FIFTY

Fashion is not something
that exists in dresses only.
Fashion is in the sky,
in the street,
fashion has to do with ideas,
the way we live,
what is happening.

Coco Chanel

DRESSING
NIFTY
AFTER FIFTY

The Definitive Guide to a
Simple, Stylish Wardrobe

Corinne Richardson

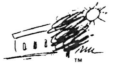

Willcott & Corn Books
Saint Louis, Missouri

DRESSING NIFTY AFTER FIFTY
The Definitive Guide to a Simple, Stylish Wardrobe

By Corinne Richardson

10 digit ISBN 0-9786636-0-8
13 digit ISBN 978-0-9786636-0-5

Library of Congress Control Number 2006928578

Book design: Peggy Nehmen, www.n-kcreative.com
Illustrations: Shelley Dieterichs, www.goodbuddynotes.com
Copy editing and indexing: Christine Frank, www.christinefrank.com

Printed in the United States of America

Published by:
Willcott & Corn Books
Post Office Box 9279
St. Louis, MO 63117 USA

*In memory of my mother
and for all women who are
determined to look their best*

Acknowledgments

I want to express my appreciation to my family and friends for their moral support, encouragement, and love.

I also want to thank the following people who have contributed to making this book possible:

Bobbi Linkemer for her enthusiasm, professional input, publishing know-how, and suggestions.

Jim Goodman for his precise editorial comments and ability to spot inconsistencies.

Christine Frank for her excellent copy editing and indexing.

Peggy Nehmen for the wonderful book design.

Shelley Dieterichs for the fantastic illustrations and cover.

Peggy Shrum and Adrienne Fairbanks for suggesting the perfect title to this book.

Annette Heller and Tom Duda for their legal expertise and practical advice.

Maria Darling and Amy Sundquist who helped me develop elegant, yet sensible taste in clothes.

Marcella Widdoes, Linda Wheatley, Adrienne Fairbanks, Greg Hoffmann, Marie Dargan, Louise Hall, Nancy Sachar, Rita Fineberg, and Pernella Cooper for expressing faith in me and the wisdom of this book.

And most importantly, Jim, my talented, loyal, and patient son; Jenni, my lovely daughter-in-law; and Katherine, my adorable granddaughter for being part of my life.

Contents

Disclaimer

Although *Dressing Nifty After Fifty* has been carefully edited, there may be some inadvertent inaccuracies, grammatical errors, and other mistakes.

Dressing Nifty After Fifty is designed to provide limited information about wardrobes for women. For more information on this and related subjects, consult the references listed in Appendix 1 and the many other books available to the public on the subjects of fashion, beauty and grooming, and aging.

Be advised and aware that none of the following named persons and entities, either individually or collectively, assume or have any responsibility, duty, obligation, or liability for any loss or damage caused or alleged to have been caused by the information provided in this book: the author, Corinne Richardson L.L.C., Willcott & Corn Books, and/or all persons and entities involved in the writing, editing, design, indexing, illustration, printing, and production of this book.

About the author

Corinne Richardson has studied fashion and design all her life, with particular interest in color and how clothing decisions affect the way people treat one another. Her other passion is the voluntary simplicity movement.

Corinne is an attorney. During her employment for thirty-one years as Chief Legal Advisor for the St. Louis County Family (Juvenile) Court, she helped simplify and organize the Court's complex administrative and legal procedures.

In 1997, Corinne took early retirement to start two consulting companies dedicated to helping people simplify their homes and businesses by minimizing their personal possessions and organizing the remainder. Her recommendations incorporate the principles of organization, interior arrangement, personal property appraisal, and Feng Shui.

In addition to her law degree, Corinne holds a Master's Degree (M.V.S.) in appraisal of property. She uses her knowledge about the fair market value of personal possessions in advising her clients about what to keep and ways to get rid of items no longer of value.

To keep current with design trends, Corinne completed a course of study with the Interior Arrangement and Design Association (IADA). She is also an avid student of Feng Shui, the Chinese art of placement, having studied with James Allyn Moser, Seann Xenja, and world-renowned Feng Shui Grand Master Professor Thomas Lin Yun. She was featured in the television special "Faith on Fox" for her Feng Shui work in homes and businesses.

In 2000, Corinne founded Corinne Richardson L.L.C. to consolidate her consulting businesses and expand her services to include ways to minimize, plan, and organize a wardrobe.

Corinne's background and hands-on experience have come together in *Dressing Nifty After Fifty*, the quintessential guide for any woman who wants an easy, simple, and sophisticated way to dress that doesn't rob her sanity or her pocketbook.

Preface

Make the best of your prime-time years

This book is for any woman who wants to create a simple, suitable, and stylish wardrobe for her prime-time years.

Perhaps you are fortunate and already know how to assemble the ideal wardrobe. For me, it has been a real challenge.

I am the only person I know who is greeted by name at the post office. Why? Because that's where I went, for many years, to return most of the clothes I bought over the Internet. And I didn't just confine myself to the Internet; I also shopped the boutiques and the malls.

Even though I was a first-class shopper, I was still confronted with that eternal mystery — a closet full of clothes and nothing to wear.

When I calculated a few years ago that the amount of clothes I owned was increasing each year by geometric proportions, I finally made the decision to get real about my wardrobe. Although part of me wanted to just keep on buying more, I simply was tired of owning so many clothes; I hated to open my closet door and see all my pretty clothes crammed together, some with their price tags still on, waiting to be worn. I became determined to have a closet with only those clothes that were suitable for all my lifestyle needs and, at the same time, fashionable and up-to-date.

My challenge was to develop an effective, easy way to figure out exactly what clothes I needed and how to be in style without sacrificing comfort and fit. After some painful years of many trials and errors, I came up with a foolproof system to create a simple, suitable, and stylish wardrobe for myself.

And so can you! If you follow the step-by-step process outlined in this book, you too can have the perfect wardrobe that takes you anywhere for any occasion.

The material is presented in a certain order to

provide easy-to-follow steps for you to create, develop, and maintain your perfect wardrobe.

To give you an overview of both the ideas presented and the process used, here is a brief summary of each chapter.

In Chapter 1 you are advised of the many benefits of creating a simple wardrobe and that fashion is about being comfortable — both physically and mentally — in what you wear.

Chapter 2 gets you started with three easy steps: (1) Buy a notebook to jot down specific ideas and strategies outlined in this book; (2) Make a commitment to a new look that is simple and stylish, while age appropriate; and (3) List your usual activities during a typical 14-day period. This last step is key to developing a wardrobe that meets all your lifestyle needs.

Chapter 3 acquaints you with the different quintessential styles of clothing; Chapter 4 shows you how to identify your particular body shape, the clothing styles that flatter you, and the styles to avoid; and Chapter 5 provides you with many tips and tricks to fool the eyes into seeing you as thinner and taller.

Chapter 6 advises you to limit your color choices to black, brown, and charcoal gray for your basic skirts, pants, and suits. At this point you may think your new look will be drab and boring. Just wait. Chapter 7 shows you how to identify and choose your best colors for blouses, sweaters, jackets, blazers, tunics, other tops, and scarves in order to add spice to your outfits. This chapter also explains when you should wear only two colors at one time, and offers advice on ways to change your image with color.

Chapter 8 outlines the different types of shoes to wear for particular occasions and the sure-fire way to test whether the shoes you are considering buying are comfortable and fit properly.

In Chapter 9, you'll discover the secrets to choosing the right handbag and belts, how to add some pizzazz with your scarves, and what basic pieces of jewelry you should own.

With this background information in mind, you will be ready to take your first concrete step towards creating your perfect wardrobe. You're advised to start with a clean slate; that is, to follow the steps outlined in Chapter 10 to clean out your closet and organize what remains.

Next, by using the process outlined in Chapter 11, you'll be able to identify and adopt what you like to wear as your private and public dress codes or uniforms. Be sure to take a look at the suggested outfits for special occasions.

Chapter 12 describes how to put together all the information you've gathered from the first eleven chapters to create your ideal wardrobe — on paper. To make the process easier, two hypothetical wardrobes, together with 14-day plans, are included.

Chapter 13 shows you exactly how to make your dream wardrobe, which you just outlined on paper, a reality. Learn how to integrate your present wardrobe with your future plans, fill in the blank spaces, and make sure you buy and wear clothes that flatter and fit you.

Chapter 14 takes you on a shopping trip and shows you how to make wise investments while buying trendy pieces on the cheap, and how to make shopping fun and productive.

You'll want to be mindful of your hands, face, and hair and follow the advice offered in Chapter 15. For example, be most careful in your purchase of eyeglasses, as your eyes are what people notice first when they look at your face.

To celebrate your new look, take a trip and travel light with the simple 10-day wardrobe detailed in Chapter 16.

And, most importantly, stay gorgeous as time goes with the sage advice offered in Chapter 17.

As for now, just turn to the next page to get started on the path to creating your own simple, stylish, and personalized wardrobe.

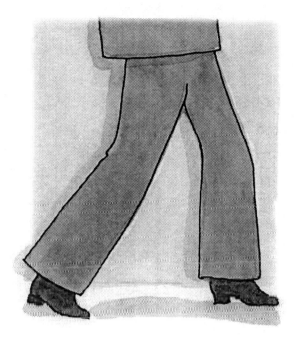

1

Put your best foot forward

Fashion is personal. It's about being comfortable — both physically and mentally — in what you wear. It's as much about how you feel when you look in the mirror as it is about how you look to others.

This book is not about owning it all. It's about creating a simple wardrobe that is suitable, stylish, and looks wonderful on you. Isn't that what we all want?

Private and public image

How you dress says a lot about you — as a reflection of how you feel about yourself and as an invitation to be treated in a certain way by others.

When I put the time and effort into looking as good as I can, I feel better. As my Grandmother Minnie Richardson used to say to me, "You've done yourself proud."

I have also learned that the clothing I wear sends out a message about me, whether I intend it to or not, and affects the way others respond to me. I think part of that phenomenon is that others treat us in the same way we treat ourselves.

A few years ago, I facilitated a discussion group of men and women ranging in age from about 50 to 75. I called the group "prime-time retirement."

When I started the group, I couldn't help but notice that quite a few people wore Bermuda shorts, worn-out tennis shoes, and old T-shirts, usually with some sort of writing on the front. I decided to ask those "casual dressers" to participate in an experiment for the next month.

I asked them to wear the following dress code whenever they left their houses: full-length jeans; plain pants or khakis; plain, white T-shirts; moccasins or walking shoes; and nice-looking navy, black, tweed, plaid, or madras blazers. Then, I asked them to notice how the general pubic responded to them. This would include grocery store clerks, salespeople, filling station attendants, and neighbors.

At the next meeting those casual dressers reported that, much to their surprise, they were treated with more kindness, assistance, friendliness, and, most importantly, with more respect than they had thought possible.

Perfect time for a simple wardrobe

Even though those casual dressers in the prime-time retirement discussion group changed their appearance, they were still asking these basic questions: Who am I? Where am I now? What do I want out of life? What are my priorities? Where am I going?

You too may be grappling with those same issues even though you are still working (full-time or part-time), starting a home-based business, recently retired and trying to figure out what you want to do next, volunteering your time, or pursuing a project or hobby.

Whatever your lifestyle or whatever changes you may be contemplating, now is the perfect time to simplify your life so you have the time and energy for the people you want to be with and the things you want to do. A wonderful way to begin is to simplify your wardrobe.

Benefits to a simple wardrobe

Perhaps you're wondering about the benefits of a simple wardrobe. Personally, I have never been able to make any changes in my life unless I knew upfront what the benefits to me would be. Here they are:

1. Deciding what to wear is a snap when you have a wardrobe that fits your every need. It means owning that wonderful pair of khakis or jeans that goes almost anywhere by simply changing your accessories.

2. Your closet will be organized, and you will be able to find everything because your clothes will be at a manageable level. Sometimes we have so much that we lose track of what we have. A friend of mine said that she knew she had gone too far when she counted 49 turtleneck T-shirts in her closet.

3. You'll find yourself buying fewer, but higher quality, items for your wardrobe. You can afford to splurge on that fabulous purse to carry every day. Or maybe it's about finally owning that designer trenchcoat with a zip-out lining.

4. You'll love and wear everything you own. A small wardrobe is better than a closet crowded with clothes that don't fit, that you never wear, and that you've forgotten why you bought in the first place. It's such a downer to find you've outgrown a lovely sweater with the price tag still on it.

5. You'll gain a sense of control over your life and a new freedom. No longer will you have to worry about what to wear or how you look. The less you worry about how you look, the more self-assured you'll be. The more self-assured you are, the more relaxed you'll feel. And, the more relaxed you feel, the easier your life will be and much more fun!

If you're convinced a simple wardrobe is for you, turn to the next chapter to get started with three easy steps.

Go confidently in the direction
of your dreams! Live the
life you've imagined. As you
simplify your life, the laws of
the universe will be simpler.

Henry David Thoreau

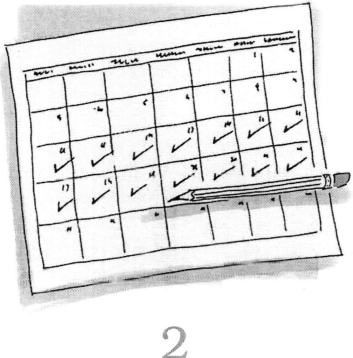

2

Get started with three easy steps

Begin with a sense of purpose about your wardrobe, and start with these three easy steps: (1) Buy a notebook to jot down specific ideas and strategies outlined in this book; (2) Make a commitment to a new look that is simple and stylish, while age appropriate; and (3) List your usual activities during a typical 14-day period. This last step is key to developing a wardrobe that meets all your lifestyle needs.

Your wardrobe notebook

Buy a notebook, and label it "My Wardrobe." Use it for only one purpose: to jot down specific ideas and strategies for creating your perfect wardrobe.

Commitment to a new you

To avoid looking like you're trying too hard, pledge to dress simply, with understated elegance. Promise yourself that you will never wear anything overtly sexy, cheap looking, or branded with a juvenile slogan.

This may be painful, but now is the time to say goodbye to three-inch and higher heels, short-shorts, mini skirts, halter-tops, novelty T-shirts, bikinis, and baby-doll outfits.

Your new look is simple and stylish, while age appropriate. This doesn't mean you have to resign yourself to blah, blah, and more blah. Instead, you'll be wearing chic, fabulous clothes with the right accessories to make your own personal statement. The next chapters will tell you how to accomplish this.

A 14-day plan

The purpose of this book is to enable you to create a wardrobe that is appropriate for your lifestyle activities. You don't want to find yourself stuck with a closet full of clothes and nothing to wear.

Just as one size does not fit all, one wardrobe does not fit all. With notebook in hand, list your usual activities during a typical 14-day period. Remember to include all activities in your plan, even if you participate in them only occasionally. Later, you will decide what styles and types of outfits are appropriate for those activities.

Knowing your lifestyle needs is an easy way to limit the quantity of clothes you own, while at the same time, ensuring that you have the right outfit for each and every occasion.

Right about now, you may be thinking: easy for you to say, difficult for me to do. Keep in mind that this step is about getting a handle on how you usually spend your time. You do not have to come up with the perfect, definitive list. If need be, you can refine the list as you proceed through later steps.

Here are two hypothetical situations to give you an idea of how to make a list of activities.

Jane Doe works full-time for five days a week for an accounting firm that expects their employees to dress in business attire Mondays through Thursdays and dress-down attire on casual Fridays. On Monday, Wednesday, and Thursday nights, she goes to a local health club after work for exercise and weight lifting, and on Tuesday and Friday nights, she relaxes with her family. On the weekend, she does household chores, hangs out with family and friends, and attends a jazz concert on one night and dines out the other night. Occasionally, she is invited to a dressy affair.

Jane's list of activities for a 14-day period looks like this:

8 Days of work (Mondays through Thursdays)

2 Days of work (dress-down Fridays)

6 Nights of exercising (Mondays, Wednesdays, and Thursdays)

4 Nights of relaxing after work (Tuesdays and Fridays)

2 Days of household chores (on weekends)

2 Additional days of relaxing (on weekends)

4 Nights of dining out/attending jazz concerts (on weekends)

1 Night at a dressy affair

The other hypothetical (outlined in the next two pages) is more complicated and is included to give you an idea of how the activities of an active lifestyle can be broken down into separate categories.

Sally Smith is recently retired from a full-time job. During a 14-day period, she volunteers her time at a local hospital for six mornings (Mondays, Wednesdays, and Fridays), and baby-sits her grandchildren for four mornings (Tuesdays and Thursdays). Her other weekday activities during a two-week period include attending two continuing education classes held on Wednesday and Friday afternoons, lunching with friends two or three times, taking long walks, going to the library, and relaxing at home whenever she can.

Sally attends monthly meetings at the Humane Society where she serves as a member of the Board of Directors. Occasionally, she meets with her banker and stockbroker.

On weekends, Sally attends religious services, does housekeeping chores such as grocery shopping and cleaning house, dines out with a movie afterwards, and relaxes the rest of the time. Whenever she can, she goes to music concerts and art exhibits. About every other month, she is invited to a formal dinner party.

When broken down into separate categories of activities, Sally's full schedule for a 14-day period looks like this:

6 Mornings of volunteer activities (Mondays, Wednesdays, and Fridays)

4 Mornings of babysitting (Tuesdays and Thursdays)

2-3 Lunches with friends

4 Afternoons of classes (Wednesdays and Fridays)

6 Afternoons (or more) of taking long walks, going to the library, and/or relaxing at home

1 Monthly meeting at Humane Society

1 Occasional meeting with banker/stockbroker

10 Nights (or more) of relaxing activities

2 Mornings/Nights of religious services (on weekends)

2 Days of housekeeping chores such as grocery shopping and cleaning (on weekends)

2 Nights of dining out and a movie (on weekends)

1-2 Nights at music concerts/art exhibits

1 Night at a formal dinner party

As stated before, the two hypothetical examples are included to give you a general idea of how to prepare your list of activities for a 14-day period.

Do not try to make your list perfect, down to the

very last detail. The idea is to provide you with a general idea of the kinds of activities in which you regularly participate. You should not spend more than 30 minutes on this step.

Finally, consider whether your activities change radically during the year. If so, you will need an additional 14-day plan or plans.

For example, if you are a teacher and you teach for nine to ten months and are on summer break for two to three months, you need two different 14-day plans: one for work and one for the summer break. The same is true if you have a seasonal job, such as a landscape planner.

Now that you have completed your list of different activities, your next step is to start thinking about what kinds of outfits you wear or want to wear for each activity.

To help you determine the types and styles of clothes for your perfect wardrobe, the next three chapters describe in detail the basic styles of clothing, how clothes can enhance your body shape, and ways to look thinner and taller.

But first, let me send you a high-five for completing your journey this far.

I base my fashion taste
on what doesn't itch.

Gilda Radner

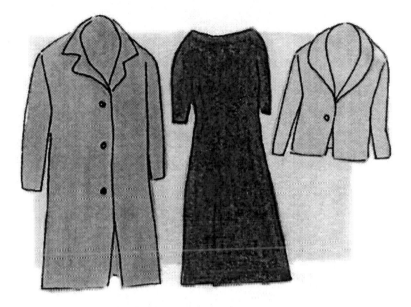

3

Consider these different styles

Clothing comes in a variety of types and styles. Read the following brief descriptions of different types of clothing and start to select the ones you want to include in your perfect wardrobe.

Skirt suits

Nothing says, "I've got it all together" as much as a skirt suit. Regardless of your lifestyle, you need at least one.

The publication in the late 1970s of *The Woman's Dress for Success Book*[1] by John Molloy caused a revolution. Women everywhere were rushing out to buy skirt suits, high-neck blouses, and small floppy scarves.

But starting in the 1990s, many in the work force abandoned this formalized style of dress for a more casual look. Just how casual depended on the particular business or profession.

Keep in mind that what is acceptable today may be unacceptable tomorrow. Even so, skirt suits are always appropriate to wear to funerals, weddings, formal luncheons, graduation ceremonies, religious services, and business functions.

Concerning the length of the skirt, somewhere around the knee is a safe look. If you don't have the greatest knees (few do), a skirt that falls just below the knee is perfect. Be sure it hangs straight on your body and the hemline is even.

The wisdom of wearing a skirt suit for formal business occasions applies not only to the work environment, but also to any situation where a mature, competent, and intelligent image is desired or beneficial. You never know when your appearance

1. John T. Molloy, *The Woman's Dress for Success Book* (New York: Warner, 1977).

might just tip the scales in your favor when decisions are being made that might affect your future. An example would be a meeting between you, your lawyer, and the IRS.

Moreover, wearing a skirt suit can be a compliment to the person you are meeting. It is a sign of respect when you have gone to the trouble to dress in an appropriate manner.

Here's the type of outfit you should wear when you have a business appointment with your banker, stock broker, lawyer, the IRS, or someone like Donald Trump: a charcoal gray or black suit with a skirt that falls slightly below the knee, a tailored blouse, a black belt, flesh-colored hose, and black, low- or mid-heel pumps. Confine your jewelry to a watch, stud earrings, and either a necklace or pin.

Complement this outfit with a black handbag and a slim portfolio for important papers. If you decide to use a larger tote bag instead of a portfolio, don't make the mistake of carrying a handbag at the same time. You can put your personal items in a small purse that is tucked inside the larger tote bag.

Extra skirts

There are many occasions when you might welcome the

option of wearing a skirt instead of a pantsuit or dress. For that reason, consider adding a few extra skirts to your wardrobe. Chose only those styles of skirts that flatter your body shape and make you look thin and tall (more on this in the next two chapters).

Pantsuits

Regardless of your age or lifestyle, a pantsuit is appropriate for most occasions. Can you think of one woman who doesn't own at least one pantsuit?

Today, it is acceptable to wear a pantsuit to work in most businesses and professions. You can never go wrong if you follow the dress code of successful women in your line of work or activity. For example, if you are a part-time or full-time volunteer, observe the dress code of other volunteers serving in the same or similar capacity as you.

Try to own at least one three-piece suit consisting of pant, skirt, and jacket. You can pair the jacket with either the pant or skirt to have the perfect suit for almost any occasion or situation.

Extra pants

You'll want to own a variety of extra pants. Make sure that all your extra pants can be worn with one of your blazers or suit jackets. Always think outfit.

Also keep in mind that "cute" should no longer be an adjective that describes any item of clothing you own, including your pants. This is your time to have a wardrobe that's chic and sophisticated. For that reason, regarding your choice of fabric for pants, say "no" to prints, flowers, or any kind of pattern that looks cute. Say "yes" to solid colors and pinstripes.

Here's a pant that is timeless and flattering for almost all figure types: a simple, flat-front, solid-colored pant with a center zipper. The next two chapters will help you choose the styles of pants that fit your body shape and make you look thin and tall.

Jeans and khakis

Jeans and khakis are the soul of your casual wardrobe. There are those times when nothing else will do except a fabulous pair of jeans or khakis.

If you find a brand and style in denim jeans that look good on you, buy several pair in different colors, including at least one pair in a dark navy wash for a slim and dressy look.

Khakis are a great alternative to jeans and are available in different styles and shades of tan or beige. The fact that khakis are appropriate for different activities makes them a basic item in your new, streamlined wardrobe.

Keep in mind that both jeans and khakis look great when paired with jackets from your pant and skirt suits. For a slightly dressy and balanced look, wear dark-colored shoes when you wear a light-colored pant with a dark-colored jacket or top. For example, black shoes balance an outfit of tan khakis and a black or charcoal gray jacket.

T-shirts

Hands down, a T-shirt is the most versatile piece in your wardrobe. It is indispensable for absolutely everything: socializing, work, exercise, and even sleeping. T-shirts are also the easiest way to stay in style. All you have to do is buy a couple in the latest fashion colors.

Buy inexpensive T-shirts, as they can look tired and limp after a few years. When you find a make or name brand of T-shirts that looks great on you and doesn't break the bank, buy several in different colors.

A typical T-shirt is made of cotton and may have some stretch added. Don't make the mistake of squeezing yourself into a too-tight T-shirt, which, more likely than not, will draw attention to any extra body fat. Instead, wear T-shirts that skim your body and are not too loose or too tight. When you want a fitted look, you can knot your T-shirt in the back or tuck it in your pant or skirt.

Don't be caught in public in a T-shirt with the sleeves rolled up or with juvenile or outlandish slogans, trim, or decorations splashed across the front. Instead, keep your T-shirts plain, and add a fabulous necklace, pendant, or pin.

If you find a sequined T-shirt, grab it. You can wear it with anything — even your jeans.

Blouses

Blouses are a clothing staple. You'll want to own at least one in a flattering version of white. Your choices are bright white, off-white, soft white, ivory, cream, eggshell, or oyster. Decide which white looks best on you and stick with it.

For versatility, consider also owning a blouse in a pinstripe and one in a flattering color that has a white collar and cuffs.

With your pant and skirt suits, you can create an individual look with blouses in traditional prints or patterns, stripes, irregular weaves, and bright colors. For a dressier look that can add spice to your life, try a lace-trimmed camisole with a plain pant or skirt suit.

You can also experiment with combining different textures. For example, a heavy linen blouse lends a nice touch to a wool suit, and a floral or paisley blouse appears avant-garde when worn with pinstriped pants.

Sweaters

Choose your sweaters wisely, as they may last forever. Wear only sweaters with necklines that flatter you. Find your best necklines from this list of styles: v-neck, crew, round, tank, boat neck, turtleneck, mock-turtleneck, cowl, and scrunch.

Silk and cashmere sweaters feel luxurious. The only disadvantage is that most must be dry-cleaned or hand-washed.

A lightweight cardigan sweater in off-white or one of your best colors comes in handy in warmer weather. It can be worn alone or with a T-shirt, slung around the shoulders, or hand-carried in case you need it.

Invest in at least one medium-weight, year-round sweater set in a color that is always in style, like coral or turquoise. Regardless of your body type or height, a flattering length for a sweater set is just below the waist.

Blazers

You can always pair the jackets of your suits with your extra pants and skirts. Even so, you should invest in a few fantastic-looking blazers.

There's no end to the different styles and types of blazers available today. If you're going for a lean look, restrict your selection to single-breasted blazers. On the other hand, if you are slender, tall, and small-breasted, see how you look in a double-breasted blazer. Be sure that whatever style you choose, it is slightly tapered to avoid a mannish look.

You may not be able to resist owning a wool blazer in a light color. Just remember that you will be dry-cleaning it often. Instead, consider a light-colored blazer in a washable fabric, such as a blend of rayon or cotton with spandex.

For a sporty look, you should have no trouble finding the latest style in motorcycle, barn, and windbreaker jackets; pea coats; and parkas. Many of them are available in different textures and patterns, such as herringbone tweed, Black Watch plaid, floral, paisley, and sharkskin.

If you must have a leather blazer, go with basic black. If you're careful, you may never have to dry-clean it. Better still: put your money in a washable suede blazer.

While I don't recommend investing in a navy blazer, you may want to own one to wear with your charcoal gray pants and skirts, and your khakis. However, you can't wear a navy blazer with blue jeans because wearing all blue is too coordinated for a chic, sporty look. That principle also applies to denim jackets, which should not be worn with matching denim pants. Instead, pair your denim jackets with your black pants or khakis.

Rather than spending your money on a navy blazer, I recommend that you buy a fabulous black blazer, which is versatile, looks rich and classy, and can be worn year-round.

If you are of average height or taller, you may want to consider a poncho or shawl as a snappy addition to your wardrobe. Either can be worn as a substitute for a jacket or blazer, or as outerwear in chilly weather.

The little black dress

Your "little black dress" can be short-sleeved or sleeveless and is most flattering in a slim, A-line shape. Just imagine how wonderful you will look when you add your pearls, á la Chanel.

Best of all, you can wear your little black dress anywhere by simply changing your jacket. For example, a black knee-length dress looks fabulous with a lightweight black gabardine jacket that falls slightly below the waist. Now, exchange that jacket for a cropped blue-jean jacket or black sharkskin blazer. Talk about casual chic!

Changing your accessories is another way to alter the formality of an outfit based on your little black dress. For example, for casual occasions, wear sandals and hoop earrings. For the office or a luncheon, complete your outfit with a simple pin, stud earrings, scarf, black pumps, and a tote bag.

For dressier times, carry a clutch or purse with a short handle, and dazzle the crowd with a gold pin, charm bracelet, and black pumps. When you dress for an even fancier affair, sling a jewel-encrusted purse over your shoulder, and add glamour with a pearl necklace, pearl earrings, brooch or pin on your shoulder, and black satin pumps.

Extra dresses

Dresses come in a wide variety of styles. Check out your fashion magazines to see what's hot. However, you may not want to invest a lot of money in a dress in this season's cutting-edge style, since it will look dated next year.

Since a dress is a combination of a blouse and skirt, consider what necklines and skirt styles look good on you to know what types of dresses will flatter you.

Conservative clothes

As mentioned under skirt suits, you'll need a few conservative, classic clothes for somber occasions such as funerals, weddings, formal luncheons, graduation ceremonies, religious services, and business functions. Always choose your outfit based on what is generally considered acceptable attire for the particular occasion.

Dressy clothes

If you go out in the evening, or attend cocktail, holiday, or other types of parties, you'll need a dressy outfit or two.

Think outfit, rather than separate pieces. For example, you might combine an ivory or black shell with a fancy jacket and black pants (made of silk for warm weather or wool for cold weather). Or, you could start with a plain black pantsuit and add a silk shell or T-shirt with crystal piping around the neck.

If you love the color beige, here's your outfit: a

monochromatic combination of beige palazzo or wide pants in a silk fabric with a matching or tonal cashmere sweater and flowing scarf.

A word of caution: don't spend a lot of money on a fancy outfit if you're only going to wear it a few times. Should you need to buy a ball gown, keep it simple, and change your accessories to update your appearance.

Trenchcoat or raincoat

You can never have too many raincoats. Here are some of your choices: full-length, knee-length, trench, and balmacaan (a loose-fitting style usually with raglan sleeves).

For adaptability, consider a raincoat in three-quarters or seven-eighths length to double as a topcoat or long jacket.

Your coat may have a hood, epaulets, or belt. There are several ways to wear a belt: knotted instead of belted, hanging open and free, or pulled through the side loops and buckled in back.

While beige is the classic color for a trenchcoat or raincoat, it's fun to own several ones in different colors, lengths, and styles. It's even better when you find ones that are washable and inexpensive.

I haven't always followed the "inexpensive" part of that last sentence. About ten years ago, I decided that I just had to have a well-made, all-weather trenchcoat. After months of searching and armed with my yearly budget allotment for clothing, I bought a long, double-breasted Burberry trenchcoat with a removable wool lining. Whenever I wear it, I feel very elegant. That's what makes the coat worth every nickel.

Winter or all-weather coat

If you want your winter or all-weather coat to be appropriate for all occasions, it should be plain; that is, without a belt, epaulets, or trim.

A simple, all-weather coat in three-quarters or seven-eighths length looks modern over pants, and over both short and long skirts. It is no longer a fashion crime to wear a coat that is shorter than the skirt underneath.

Your coat should fit loosely over all your clothes. Before you purchase a new coat, take your bulkiest jacket or blazer with you. If the coat slides over that jacket or blazer without pulling, you'll know that the coat will go over all of your other jackets and blazers. Remember to take a look in a three-way mirror to be sure that the coat lies flat across the back and that the overall fit is not too snug.

If you can't find a coat you like, consider having a dressmaker make you a lightweight topcoat. A few years ago, I saw a gorgeous ultrasuede fabric in chocolate brown on sale. I found a dress pattern in a loose-fitting, long, topcoat style with a notched collar and pockets. I had the fabric store recommend a dressmaker, and away I went with my fabric and pattern in hand. The coat turned out even better than I had imagined; it's machine-washable and should last a lifetime.

With that last bit of advice about coats, turn now to the next chapter to identify your body shape, and find out which styles will flatter your figure and which styles you should avoid.

Clothes should look as if a woman was born into them. It is a form of possession, this belonging to one another.

Geoffrey Beene

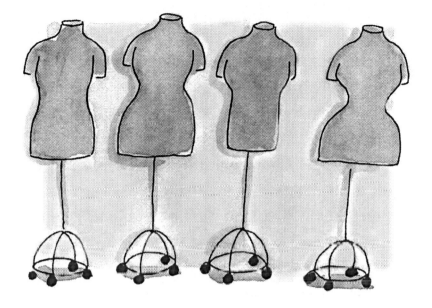

4

Enhance your body shape
with clothes

When your wardrobe consists of only those clothes that flatter your body shape, you will have changed your looks from so-so to fantastic. However, first you must reconcile yourself to the fact that you can't wear all styles of clothing.

How many times have you gone through this scenario? You see an outfit that looks smashing on your closest friend. You search and, fortunately, or so you think, you find a similar outfit in a store. You try it on and look in the mirror. You can't remember a time when you looked worse or felt more uncomfortable.

Don't despair. The reason the outfit didn't look the same on you as it did on your friend is because the two of you have different body shapes. Clothes that look good on her may not look good on you and vice versa. Instead of trying to transform yourself into a clone of your friend, concentrate on identifying your unique body shape and the clothing details that flatter you.

In order to analyze what looks good on you, consider the four basic body shapes, commonly referred to as the rectangle, pear, inverted triangle, and hourglass. Be aware that those four shapes are not related to your height, weight, or bra or clothing size. Instead, they are related to the total or overall impression created by your figure.

Look at your body in a full-length mirror. What do you see — a rectangle, a pear, an inverted triangle, or an hourglass?

The rectangle

The rectangle shape describes the woman with a straight or boyish build. Think Audrey Hepburn. You are a rectangle shape if you consistently buy both the tops and bottoms of pant and skirt suits in the same size; you also like garments that are described as being straight, such as straight skirts or pants with straight legs.

You look your best in clothes that mimic, rather than contrast with, your body shape. Choose boxy, geometric, straight-falling clothes, such as pants with straight legs.

Don't try to add curves by wearing rounded shoulder pads, gathered pleats, or scoop necklines. You probably have never met a belt you liked. Put a belted winter coat on you, and you feel like you've gained ten pounds. Unless you have long, slim legs, chances are that you also don't look great in boot-cut or full-cut pants.

Here are some clothing details that flatter the rectangle shape:

- Necklines that are square, ruched, stand-up, boat, jewel, V, or mandarin

- Turtlenecks

- Set-in sleeves

- Shoulder pads that are straight (sometimes identified as square)

- Pockets that are square or slashed
- Skirts or pants with no pleats at all or pleats that are stitched or pressed down
- Pant legs that are straight or slightly tapered
- Jacket lapels and blouse collars that are sharp, notched, or pointed
- Jackets that are loose or fitted
- Hemlines that are straight

The pear

The pear shape describes you if your body below your waist is broader than your body above your waist. You have a pear shape if you consistently buy pants and skirts in one size, and jackets and other tops in a smaller size.

Your goal is to draw attention to your upper body in order to balance your figure. Widen your shoulders with shoulder pads, boat necks, and horizontal details. If you are small-breasted, consider pockets and details at the bust line.

You can also emphasize the top half of an outfit with eye-catching details, such as an embroidered jacket, a vest, a smashing pin, or scarf.

Avoid belted and cropped styles, drawstring pants, clingy fabrics, flap or patch pockets, and anything that hits you at the widest part of your hips.

Your best look may be light-colored tops with dark-colored skirts or pants.

Here are some clothing details that flatter the pear shape:

- Clothes that are loose-fitting
- Necklines that are wide, sailor, winged, boat, halter, V, cowl, or crew
- Turtlenecks, if not overpowering
- Cap sleeves
- For knit fabrics, shoulder pads that are rounded; for other fabrics, shoulder pads that are straight (sometimes identified as square)
- Empire waists
- Skirts that are A-line, gored, or flared
- If flattering, skirts that stop at the knee
- Pants and skirts that are pin-striped
- Pants that have side-zippers and flat-fronts
- Pant legs that are straight or slightly wide

- Jacket lapels and blouse collars that are peaked, notched, wide, or winged

- Jackets that are double-breasted or shirt-style

The inverted triangle

The inverted triangle shape is the reverse of the pear shape and describes you if your body above your waist is broader than your body below your waist. You know your figure is shaped like an inverted triangle if you consistently buy pants and skirts in one size, and jackets and other tops in a larger size.

Your objective is to bring your figure into proportion. Generally, you look good in most styles, as long as the top half of your body is minimized.

In other words, avoid anything that emphasizes your upper body. Examples are flap pockets at the breast; tight or stretch T-shirts or sweaters; and jackets, blouses, and tunics that are cropped, waist-high, or double-breasted.

Raglan sleeves for a sweater or blouse are flattering as long as you are not full-breasted; if you are, try instead a sweater or blouse with a wide-open neckline and sleeves that are either set-in or have no shoulder seams.

Although you have to be careful to get the right look,

consider wearing dark-colored tops over light-colored skirts or pants.

Here are some clothing details that flatter the inverted triangle shape:

- Semi-fitted styles
- Anything with an open collar
- Necklines that are scoop, cowl, or V
- No shoulder pads
- Tops that are slightly fitted with high V-necklines
- Jacket lapels and blouse collars that are small, peaked, notched, or plain shawl
- Jackets and tops that end at mid-hip
- Jackets that are single-breasted and close just below the bust line

The hourglass

The hourglass shape is like an X shape. Think Marilyn Monroe. You have an hourglass figure if you consistently buy clothes that emphasize your waistline and your curves, such as nipped-in or belted jackets.

As with the rectangle shape, look for clothes that mimic and repeat the lines of your body. An example would be a jacket with a shawl lapel and rounded hemline rather than a jacket with a peaked lapel and straight hemline.

Choose fabrics that skim, rather than cling to, your curves. Don't try to create straight lines, and avoid boxy styles, square necklines, pleated skirts, and geometric styles. Just go with your curvy figure.

Here are some clothing details that flatter the hourglass shape:

- Necklines that are round, scoop, draped, ruffled, and cowl
- Sleeves that are drop-shoulder or raglan
- Shoulder pads that are rounded
- Pockets that are flap, rounded, or set-in
- Waists that are nipped-in
- Pants and skirts with pleats that are soft, gathered, and eased
- Pant legs that are boot-cut or wide
- Jacket lapels and blouse collars that are rounded, shawl, or curved
- Slighted fitted jackets with well-defined waistlines and rounded hemlines

Now that you've identified your particular body shape, read on to learn how to fool the eyes into seeing your shape narrowed and stretched to a thinner, taller you.

Fashion is the science of appearances, and it inspires one with the desire to seem rather than to be.

Michel de Montaigne

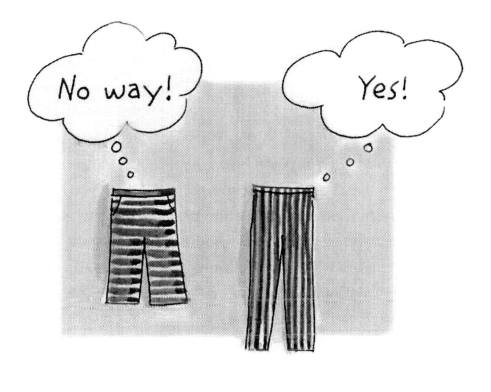

5

Look thinner and taller

While you can't change your proportions, there are many ways to create a thinner, taller you.

A good foundation

Be sure your undergarments do the best for you. I cannot emphasize enough the importance of a well-fitting bra that offers you the most support. When you go to a store, find a saleswoman to ensure you are wearing the right size. A good bra can take years off your appearance.

If you are tempted to buy a very fancy lace bra, remember to try it on with a sweater. You don't want to look like your boobs need ironing.

At a minimum, buy one white bra, two ivory or skin-tone bras, and one black bra. Add a push-up bra if you wear garments with low necklines.

If you wear lots of trousers and pants, rarely will you need to wear a slip. Just in case, though, it never hurts to have two camisoles, one in ivory and one in black; if you wear dresses of thin fabrics, include one full-slip in ivory and one in black. You also need a few half-slips, at least one that stops at your knee and another that is mid-calf.

Don't overlook your hose. They can be important to your overall appearance. Consider control-top pantyhose or body shapers to trim and mold your body.

General rules

Thin and tall go together. If you concentrate on looking thinner, you will automatically look taller.

Your clothes must fit your body and not bag, sag, or gag. Don't even think about shoving yourself into something that's too tight and is physically miserable.

At the same time, wearing over-sized clothes will make you look sloppy and bigger than you are. Strike a balance between style and comfort, and be sure your clothes are in proportion to your weight and height.

Don't be held hostage by the size of the garment. Those smile lines in your pants are telling you to try a larger size. Just say thank you and move on.

Sometimes you will need to buy different-size tops and bottoms. Or, even if you are of average height, you might find you need petite-size pants to fit a short waist or rise.

Proportion is everything. Think long over short and short over long. Translated, that means, as a general rule, in order to look thinner and taller, wear a long jacket with a short skirt or pant and a short jacket with a long or full skirt or pant.

Moreover, if you are short and wearing a long jacket over a short skirt, be sure to wear one-inch or higher heels to compensate for your height. Otherwise, the long jacket will end up making you look shorter than you are.

Shoulder pads are another wonderful way to bring your figure into proportion. You'll look a lot better with a sleeve that is draped over, rather than glued to, your arm. Be sure all your shoulder pads are removable so you can always wear whatever thickness is in current style.

As recommended in other chapters, you can begin to get a more exact impression of what works for your figure if you always check out your outfit in a full-length mirror. And don't forget to use another mirror so you can see the back of your outfit.

Ways to look thinner

Omit the word horizontal from your fashion vocabulary. Think vertical.

Wear clothes made of fabrics that skim over your body, rather than cling for dear life. Bulky fabrics add pounds. A fisherman's sweater can be gorgeous, but maybe not on you. The same goes for shiny, fuzzy, and elaborately embossed garments. Ditto for lots of texture.

During the colder months, stick to lightweight fabrics, such as gabardine, thin knits, silk, and rayon blends. In warmer weather, look for denim, polyester, and linen and cotton blends.

Color is another way to slenderize your looks. Try wearing tonal colors — lighter and darker shades of the same color. This works well with your basic grays and browns. Another technique is to combine different colors, which are of the same depth, such as light aqua with light brown. To look your thinnest, mix subtle medium or dark colors. For example, try medium blue with medium chocolate brown, or try charcoal gray with black.

If your stomach and hips are not as flat as you'd like, think twice before buying anything that accentuates them, such as very narrow pants and bias-cut skirts or dresses. Instead, look for looser garments made in fabrics with some stretch.

If you are unhappy with the size of your waist, you might like the look of pants and skirts with no waistbands or slightly dropped waists. For casual occasions, try this outfit: dark pantsuit with a light-colored T-shirt or blouse that hangs loose instead of tucked-in, falls straight, and is longer than and shows beneath the hemline of the jacket.

Flat-front pants and skirts with elastic only in the back of the waist are another easy-to-wear option. However, cover the elastic waist with a long blouse, tunic, or coordinated jacket. Without that coverage, you run the risk of looking dowdy.

Look for garments with inseam pockets. Avoid patch and flap pockets since they add inches to your hips. If the pockets in a skirt or pants do not lie flat, you can simply sew the pockets shut or take the pockets out altogether.

Ways to look taller

Anything you wear that cuts you into pieces or fails to create a vertical line will make you appear shorter. For that reason, you'll want to look with a jaundiced eye at belted outfits and pants that are cropped, wide, or cuffed. Instead, try a jacket that covers your hips with pants that are slim-cut and full-length; complete your outfit with an oblong scarf on the outside of the jacket.

Think of everything that lengthens the look of your body, such as high necklines, mandarin collars, shift dresses, monochromatic or tonal outfits, and scarves that are thin, long, and oblong.

If you are fortunate enough to have a long neck, no doubt you already know to emphasize it with big jewelry, turtlenecks, and scarves.

If, instead, you have a short neck, you can lengthen it with V- or U-shaped necklines, open collars, and long scarves. Keep your neckline free of anything, such as a choker necklace, and don't wear long, dangling, or chandelier earrings.

Color plays an important role in making you appear taller. One color, head to toe, is the easiest way to lengthen your body. For example, try black opaque hose with a short black skirt.

Also consider removing cuffs from pants, tapering the width of skirts and pant legs, and even changing the size of buttons on a jacket. In other words, do everything you can to simplify and streamline your appearance.

Your best skirts

Almost any length in skirts is acceptable in today's fashion world. That's good news since you will be able to confine your selection to only those skirts that flatter your figure.

In general, straight skirts look best when they fall just to or right below the knee, since skirts any shorter or much longer can ruin the proportion of an outfit.

Even though a pencil skirt that stops at the knee makes a neat appearance, one that ends at mid-calf can also be attractive, particularly when paired with a short jacket. Just make sure the skirt is not too tight and has a slit or kick pleat for easy walking.

A-line skirts are universally flattering. They should be narrow through the hips and flare slightly at the hem.

Wear boots if a mid-calf or longer skirt makes your

legs appear heavy. If you want to look taller, wear a long skirt with buttons from the waist to the hem to create a thin vertical line.

Fluid skirts usually have some length. A long gored skirt that swings when you walk looks carefree, particularly when combined with a twin sweater set.

One of the most attractive skirts is a pleated one. There are many styles from which to choose: pleats that are stitched down to the hip line, pressed pleats, and wide or narrow pleats. However, regardless of the style, the pleats should lie flat and fall straight down. Note that a skirt with stitched-down pleats looks best when it ends at or just below the knee.

Your best pants

Pants are the backbone of most women's wardrobes today. However, they can be extremely difficult to buy.

Today, pants come in a variety of lengths: full-length, ankle-length, cropped, Capri, and the old-fashioned pedal-pusher. Then, there are many widths in pant legs to consider: slim, full, relaxed, straight, and boot-cut. And, let's not forget some of the other choices in pants: high-rise and low-rise, tapered and straight legs, and waists that sit above, on, or below your natural waistline.

Whew! Maybe we should just wear skirts.

Well, pants are here to stay. So you'll want to concentrate on looking your best in them.

Your pants must fit all over. That means the back of the pant should fall straight. You don't want smile lines on the back of your thighs. Remember: all horizontal lines are out.

Tapered legs can make your hips look wider than they are. Instead, consider straight-cut pants with a slight break at the hemline for a long, lean look. Another way to minimize your hips is to buy pants with a yoke or small embroidery on the back pockets.

Keep in mind that pants that are too wide for your body will make you look sloppy and dumpy. A good dressmaker or tailor can tell you what widths of pants are flattering for you. You'll probably find out that there are several widths you can wear.

If you do decide to wear palazzo or wide-legged pants, be sure to choose soft fabrics that skim your body, and have them hemmed just short of the ground.

Sometimes the particular type of shoe that you wear with a pant will dictate the length of the pant. For example, flats look good with pants that are hemmed to the ankle and with full-length pants that end with a slight break over the front of the shoe.

73

Always try on new pants with all the shoes you might wear with them; and, if you need to have the pants hemmed by a dressmaker or tailor, take those shoes with you. You will have to compromise on the length of the pant if you want to wear heels of different heights.

The best thing about pants that are shorter than full-length is that they never have to be hemmed. The bad news is that you may not look good in any of the shorter styles.

Although easy to wear and in style, cropped pants may not be your friends, unless you are a tall, skinny woman. And, if you have short legs, keep in mind that your legs will be emphasized when you wear anything like cropped pants.

If you decide that you're going to wear the shorter styles of pants anyway, then at least follow this tip to lengthen your torso. Combine your shorter pants with jackets, blouses, tunics, or sweaters of the same colors as the pants.

With this chapter, you now have all the background information you need to start assembling your personalized simple wardrobe. You've taken a look at the quintessential styles of clothing, learned how to enhance your figure shape with clothes, and reviewed some of the tricks to create a thinner, taller you. Now you're ready to take the next step: ensuring that your wardrobe is simple and easy to manage by limiting your choices in basic items to the three colors of black, brown, and charcoal gray.

Our life is frittered away by detail. Simplify, simplify.

Henry David Thoreau

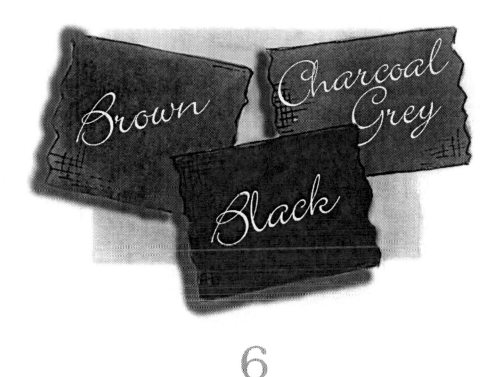

6

Stick to three colors for basics

The key to a simple wardrobe is to limit your choices. Think about the quality of what you want to own, rather than the quantity. With a smaller wardrobe, you can afford to upgrade your future purchases and, at the same time, stay within your budget.

Skirts, pants, and suits

Make the decision now to stick to the three colors of

black, brown, and charcoal gray for your basics — your skirts, skirt suits, pants, and pantsuits. Adding more colors requires more shopping, more closet space, and more money. Too many choices will ultimately lead to absolute chaos in your fashion life.

At this point, you might be wondering if limiting yourself to three colors for your basics is too boring. Just wait. You'll be adding lots of color to your outfits via your blouses, sweaters, and scarves.

Also, know that both charcoal gray or brown look great in combination with black, and don't forget the tonal look created with shades of gray or brown.

Let's now take a closer look at those three colors.

Black is fabulous as a basic color. Wearing black creates an aura of stability, style, power, grandeur, and sophistication, all at the same time. The color black is associated with depth, serious matters, the quest for justice, and the potential for development. If you like the color black, you are self-sufficient, individualistic, and protective of others; when you wear black, you will appear more social, accessible, and sexy.

Keep in mind that black looks great when paired with a myriad of colors or on its own. For a sure winner, you can never go wrong with the combination of a black suit with a white top, one of those simple outfits that spell classic, rich, and sophisticated. And, as we all know, there's nothing like the power of a simple, basic black dress.

Charcoal gray signifies the balance of black and white or resolution of conflict. It makes a less formal impression than black, yet appears business-like. Think of the color banker's gray. If you are comfortable with this color, you are practical, calm, and conservative.

Brown is the color of the earth and connotes responsibility, grounding, and a sense of nature. Wearing brown gives you an aura of grace and elegance. If you like the color brown, you are down-to-earth, loyal, and reliable with your feet "on the ground."

When shopping for basic items for your spring and summer wardrobes, look for these wonderful variations of charcoal gray and brown: medium gray, rose beige, mushroom, and dark taupe.

Color variations

There can be color variations between different garments, depending on the fabric and dye used. When combining separates, be sure to compare them in direct sunlight.

With the color black, there might be a shading or

tinge of navy, brown, purple, or gray in the black color. For that reason, you need to be careful when combining two black items made by different manufacturers or purchased at different times. The two items may not match or even blend in color, and look tacky when worn together as an outfit.

If the black in your jacket has a tinge of purple, the black in your pants should also have a tinge of purple. The two garments do not have to match exactly, but should go together or complement one other.

The same problem can also occur when you are combining two garments in brown or charcoal gray. A brown fabric can have an undertone of either yellow or gray, and a charcoal gray fabric can look as if it has green, yellow, or navy mixed with the gray.

After you have taken the time to look at your outfit in direct sunlight to ensure that the colors match or are a close blend, you may want to add a splash of color. Read the next chapter to see how.

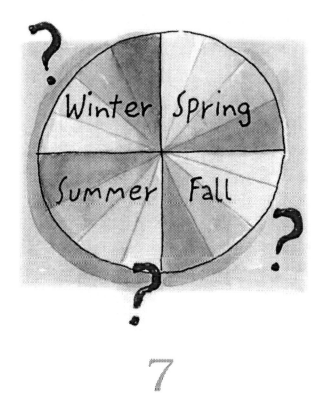

7

Add color to your outfits

Color is the spice of your wardrobe. Add color to your outfits with your blouses, sweaters, tunics, blazers, jackets, scarves, and other tops. The right color can change your outfit from dull to sharp, boring to exciting, and matronly to sophisticated.

It's amazing how the use of color can alter the way you look. For example, when you wear an item of clothing close to your face that repeats the color of your eyes, you create the look of integrity since the colors are consistent.

Think of color as having weight. You can mix vibrant colors or soft pastels of the same weight or intensity. For instance, pair bright blue with bright green or yellow, and try pale peach with beige or celedon green. You can also wear a mix of colors that, if blended together, would make another color. For example, because white mixed with black makes a charcoal color, a pair of black pants, white blouse, and a charcoal jacket looks casual, classic, and chic all at once.

As mentioned in Chapter 3, to update last year's favorite pantsuit, just make sure your blouse, shell, T-shirt, or sweater is in one of the latest fashion colors. That's the easy way to always stay in style.

Color Analysis

If you know your "color season" (winter, spring, summer, or autumn) and what colors look best on you, you have already taken a major step toward creating your perfect wardrobe. However, if you are not familiar with this concept, here's some background information to get you started.

In the early 1980s, Carole Jackson's book, *Color Me*

Beautiful[2] created a sensation. People everywhere were having "their colors done." Clothing catalogues even started to identify a particular item for sale by its "color season." For example, a suit offered in rose brown was identified as a "summer" suit and a shocking pink blouse as perfect for a "winter."

The color theories that were advanced in *Color Me Beautiful* are as valid today as when originally conceived. Here are the four seasons of color described in *Color Me Beautiful*.

Winter's colors are deep, bright, and cool (with blue undertones). Picture a cold, icy, mountaintop where the air is sharp and crisp.

Spring's colors are light, bright, and warm (with yellow undertones) like the colors painted on Easter eggs and seen on a clear spring day.

Autumn's colors are deep, muted, and warm (with yellow undertones), and reminiscent of the colors you see when the leaves start to turn gold, rust, and brown.

Summer's colors are light, muted, and cool (with blue undertones). Think of a soft summer day where everything is a blend of medium-range colors that seem to have a slight film of dust over them.

2.   Carole Jackson, *Color Me Beautiful: Discover Your Natural Beauty Through the Colors that Make You Look Great & Feel Fabulous!* (Washington, D.C.: Acropolis, 1984).

If you don't know which colors look best on you, rather than trying to figure that out on your own, consult an expert who identifies colors by seasons or some other similar system.

Most experts will test all colors on you to determine which ones are the most flattering. They may also provide color swatches for your use when shopping. However, as I found out, sales clerks do not necessarily appreciate customers using color swatches to determine if the color of an item is "right" for them.

In 1985, I took my son on a European tour for his high school graduation present. In an expensive, high-end store in London, I whipped out my colors just to make sure that the sweater I was considering buying was the right shade of blue. When the sales clerk saw what I was doing, she exclaimed: "I can't stand to see another one of those color charts; they're driving me crazy. Out! Out!" Taken aback and feeling somewhat chagrined, I quickly apologized and said I was a fashion moron who needed help wherever I could get it. Fortunately, my apology seemed to calm her down; I was then able to compare the sweater to my color swatches. I was delighted to find that the sweater was in the right shade of blue, and bought it immediately.

Colors for everyone

Everyone can wear coral, turquoise, periwinkle blue, and soft or off-white.

You may want to add the color pink to that list. Wearing the color pink next to your face is an easy way to give yourself a rosy, healthy glow. If you find that pink is not listed among the colors of your personal palette, don't despair. See how you look in apricot or a warm yellowed pink.

Individual color test

Keep in mind that the right color is the one that brings your face to life. The wrong color drains your face of any color. Here's how to test yourself to determine if a color looks good on you.

Stand in front of a full-length mirror. Wear a simple outfit in a color that looks good on you. Close your eyes. When you open your eyes, your face, not your body, should be the first thing you see. Now hold the bottom of a garment you want to test next to your face, under your chin. Close your eyes. Wait a few seconds. Open your eyes. What do you see first?

If your face pops out at you, you can safely conclude that the color you are testing is your color. If, however, your body is the first thing you see, don't wear that color! If you can't focus on either your face or your body, the color you are testing is also not for you.

You can have someone else look at you and do the color test. Whichever that person sees first — your face or body — determines whether the color is right for you.

The colors you wear should add a glow to your complexion and minimize lines and wrinkles. Why would you want to settle for anything less? Well, here's why you might.

You decide to find out if the clothes you already own are in your best colors. So you start to compare the colors of your clothes with your color swatches or perform the color test outlined above. Much to your horror, you discover that some of your clothes are not in the right colors. To make matters worse, those clothes are relatively new. You are now in what is called a "wardrobe nightmare."

Not to worry. Those not-so-flattering colors will look fine on you, as long as you wear one of your more flattering colors next to your face. For example, you have a classic navy blazer from last year, and navy next to your face does not look good. You can take a vow that, whenever you wear the navy blazer, you will also put something next to your face that is in one of your best colors. That something might be a blouse, sweater, T-shirt, or scarf.

Only two colors per outfit

When your outfit is confined to two colors, your look is balanced; everything flows together. Picture yourself in a pantsuit of one color with a blouse or sweater in a different color. Or, see how you look in pants of one color with both a T-shirt and jacket in a second color. Or, try on pants and top (blouse, T-shirt, or sweater) in one color with a jacket in a second color as an accent. Looking good just doesn't get much easier!

Conversely, if you wear more than two colors at once for any activity other than just relaxing or hanging out, you run the risk of looking as if you threw your outfit together without a thought or care. My boss once accused me of getting dressed in a closet with the lights out. I didn't make that mistake again.

When you count the number of colors in the outfit you are wearing, do not include a T-shirt, blouse, sweater, or tunic that is white or a version of white, such as off-white, soft white, ivory, cream, eggshell, or oyster. Note that parchment and oatmeal are not considered to be shades of white, since they are related to the color beige.

As an example of how to calculate the number of colors, an outfit of khaki pants, black jacket, and white T-shirt consists of two colors: khaki and black; the white T-shirt is not included.

However, white is counted as a color when it is the color of your jacket, blazer, vest, dress, pants, skirt, or pant or skirt suit. For instance, an outfit of khaki pants, black T-shirt, and white jacket consists of three colors: khaki, black, and white.

Multi–colored patterns, such as Black Watch plaid, are always considered as one separate color. This can be confusing if the pants or skirt is in one of the colors in the jacket.

For example, suppose you have an outfit consisting of a black and white plaid jacket and solid black pants. The plaid jacket stands alone as one color with the pants as the second color. To continue with this illustration, if you were wearing this outfit in a business-like setting or for a luncheon, you could wear a white blouse, shell, or T-shirt (remember, white tops aren't included in your color count). But, if you were meeting friends for a TGIF get-together, you might want take the outfit down a notch by adding more color, such as a red T-shirt, sweater, or scarf.

To re-cap, for those times when you want a casual

look, ignore the rule of only two colors at once, and wear three or more colors. To see how this works, put on a charcoal gray pantsuit with a red sweater. Your look is pulled-together and you're ready to go almost anywhere. Now, change the charcoal gray pants to black pants. Instantly, your look becomes less formal. Or, try on blue jeans, black jacket or blazer, and black T-shirt. Now switch the color of the T-shirt from black to turquoise. You've gone from sophisticated and hip to casual and relaxed.

In order to decide how many colors to wear at one time, consider the impression you want to make on the particular occasion. As always, make sure that your outfit is appropriate, chic, and stylish.

Color and Feng Shui

Feng Shui (pronounced "fung shway") is the Chinese art of placement. It is an ancient science with records dating back to the fourth century B.C.

To learn about the role and use of color in applying Feng Shui principles to surroundings and in different areas of life, consult *Living Color*[3] by Sarah Rossbach and Lin Yun. This well-written and fascinating book outlines many reasons for wearing certain colors. For

3. Sarah Rossbach and Lin Yun, *Living Color: Master Lin Yun's Guide to Feng Shui and the Art of Color* (New York: Kodansha, 1994).

example, if you want to lose weight, wear white.

The colors you choose affect others. If you want to create a certain impression or increase your fortune in a specific area, experiment by wearing a particular color. Here are a few suggestions.

Red is linked to justice, happiness, warmth (like fire), and energy. Wear red when you want to appear motivated and dynamic.

Pink is the color for the heart, and so, its association with love. If you want to attract romance into your life, choose pink as an accent color.

Purple is linked to abundance and wealth. According to an old Chinese saying, "it is so red, it is purple"[4] meaning the ultimate has been reached. Adding even a touch of purple to your outfit may open the door to a richer life.

Green stands for new beginnings, freshness, growth, and hope for the future. You may discover you are more creative when you wear green.

Blue, similar to green, symbolizes spring, and conveys a cool feeling. Dark blue or navy is particularly appropriate for serious formal occasions. Wearing blue may help you expand your knowledge.

Since you now know how to spice up your outfit

4. Rossbach, *Living Color*, 46

with color, it is time to shift to a discussion of the one item that can make or break not only your outfit, but your over-all comfort and confidence. Of course, we are talking about your shoes.

Regardless of the time you spend putting your outfit together with just the right touch of color or how gorgeous you look in the finished product, if your feet are in agony, you will be miserable.

If you think that you have to cram your feet into killer heels to look good, you are mistaken. Instead, follow the suggestions in the next chapter to combine comfort with style in your shoes. Your feet will love you forever.

Luxury must be comfortable,
otherwise it is not luxury.

Coco Chanel

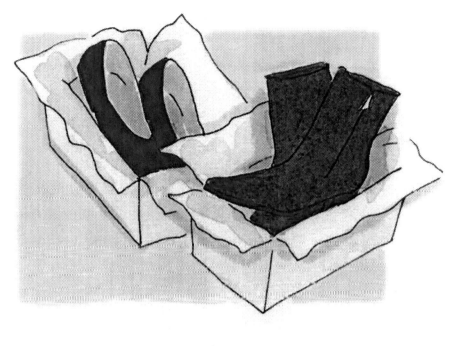

8

Combine comfort with style in your shoes

Since I'm known as a lover of shoes, I have received numerous comments, or shall I say jabs, along these lines: "I cannot believe anyone could possibly own so many pairs of shoes." And then, someone even had the gall once to add: "You don't seem to realize you can only wear one pair at a time." A low blow, but I try to remember that comment every time I go shoe shopping, one of my favorite pastimes.

Yes, there was a time when I owned over a hundred pairs of shoes. Today I would own at least that number if I could comfortably wear high heels, but I can't.

Comfort and fit

There's no getting around the fact that comfortable shoes make your life a lot easier. At the same time, shoes that are good for your feet can remind you of the ones your grandmother wore.

It's time to get real. Three-inch and higher heels look best on younger women. After your fiftieth birthday, you look silly if you try to walk in stiletto heels, otherwise known as stilts. Why risk falling, even if you can "stand" them (pardon the pun)? Thank heavens, there are plenty of low-heel shoes that are fantastic looking and available in different styles.

However, it's easy to try on a pair of shoes that looks terrific on the display rack, but not on your feet. Also, keep in mind that no good comes from buying shoes in the wrong length or width. If the salesclerk tells you the shoes will feel fine once you've broken them in, don't believe it. Here's a way to test your prospective purchase.

Buy the shoes only if you can return them for a full refund. After you get home, get out a pair of old socks. Now, put the shoes on and pull the socks on and over the shoes to completely cover and protect them. When you walk, the socks, not the soles of the shoes, will touch the floor.

After you've paraded around your home for about thirty minutes, you will know whether the shoes are comfortable. If your feet feel like you've been walking on a cloud, you can congratulate yourself on a splendid purchase. However, if your feet complain that they've been walking around in the shoes from hell, take off the socks and shoes, and return the shoes in store-bought condition for a full refund.

Safety first

If you are concerned about tripping or falling down, look for shoes with a sole made of a non-slip rubber or other gripping material. Should you buy ones with plain leather soles, you can take the shoes to a repair shop to have rubber applied to the top half of the sole. You can also safely have a lift (usually about a quarter of an inch) taken off the heel to lower the height of the shoes while leaving the balance and basic style of the shoes intact.

Guidelines for shoes to own

Buy the best shoes you can afford. The quality of your shoes can make or break an outfit.

You can never go wrong with basic black shoes; they are perfect with skirts, pants, and pant and skirt suits that are in the colors of black, charcoal gray, and brown. For variety, include a few khaki and brown shoes in your shoe wardrobe.

There's no end to the countless details that differentiate one shoe from another. You might like ones made of fake crocodile or snakeskin, or you may prefer ones with a cutout pattern or decorations such as bows or buckles. And there are always the classic spectator shoes in black or brown with white.

You can change your appearance simply by changing your shoes. For example, with a plain pantsuit, exchange low-heel pumps for sneakers or walking shoes for a completely different look.

If you work in a conservative business or profession, polish off your outfit with plain low- or mid-heel pumps. For work in a creative field, find out whether flat shoes are acceptable.

As a general rule, the shorter the skirt, the lower the heel. A plain, slim, knee-length skirt looks great with pumps that have small, tapered heels. If the skirt has a waistline that falls below your natural waist, flats are a better choice.

Wear low- to mid-heel pumps with straight or A-line skirts that fall at mid-calf or to the ankle. If you are of average height or taller, you can wear flats or no-heel boots with long, full skirts.

It can be hard to decide which pair of shoes to wear with a particular outfit. This is another instance when you should check out your appearance in a full-length mirror — the best way to decide which pair of shoes is the perfect complement to your outfit.

Here is a list of the basic styles of shoes. Read the descriptions of the different types to select the ones you need for your wardrobe:

- Black leather low- to mid-heel pumps are essential. You can do no better than low-heel shoes in the Ferragamo style, real or look-alike.

- Black leather pumps with slim or kitten heels add class to skirts, trousers, and cropped pants, and are appropriate day or night. Think Audrey Hepburn.

- Black leather mid-heel pumps with a thick heel look great with pants and trousers, and also with short or long skirts, as long as you wear opaque black hose.

- Black leather loafers and oxfords seem to be made for pants. Think Katharine Hepburn.

- Black leather flats look best with either round or pointed toes and some decoration, like a bow or tassel. A half-inch to one-inch heel on a flat makes the flat look dressier and may be more comfortable to wear. Avoid ballet slippers, if you discover they make you look shorter than you are.

- Black suede pumps and loafers are more formal in appearance than ones in leather. Other styles of dress shoes can be hard to find in low heels. The ones that look delicate or show some skin, such as slingbacks and D'Orsay (shoes that have an enclosed toe and heel, but expose the foot's arch), are your best bet.

- Silver or gold metallic flats, ballet slippers, and black satin low-heel pumps are options for formal affairs.

- Open-toed shoes and sandals look great in the summer, but only if your ankles are trim and you get regular pedicures.

- Black patent leather low-heel pumps and loafers can be worn instead of sandals and are a welcome change, year-round.

- Tennis shoes are for walking, hiking, exercise, and playing tennis. You can find some designer tennis or running shoes, but they may not be worth the high price tag.

- Walking shoes in black suede add a touch of style to full-length jeans, pants, and trousers, but look clumsy with skirts.

- Short black boots are perfect with full-length pants, but nothing else.

- Cowboy boots, clogs, espadrilles, and platforms are for casual wear only.

- Black waterproof boots for rainy and cold weather are a must.

Shoe care

When you have gone to the trouble to find shoes that are comfortable, fit your feet, and look stylish, you'll want to keep them looking as good as new. If you take proper care of your shoes, they will last for years.

Protect your new shoes with a shoe spray that is appropriate for the shoe material and store them in their original or plastic boxes.

Nothing ruins your appearance more than scratched, unpolished shoes. Be sure to periodically wax and shine your leather shoes, and brush your suede ones.

You can count on dirty hands and ruined manicures if you wait until the last minute to spit and polish your shoes. To ensure that your shoes are always ready for wear, don't put them away until you've checked them for scuffs. If they need care, you can either do so immediately or put them somewhere to remind you that they need attention.

Make sure the end tips of the heels are in good shape. If not, take them to a repair store to have the end tips replaced.

Hose and socks

There's nothing like body shapers and control-top pantyhose to improve the fit of your skirts and pants, and support hose to make the leg muscles feel like new. I know some women who have been wearing support hose ever since they were pregnant.

You can determine if a particular color of hose complements your skin tone by stretching one leg of the hose over your arm and comparing it with your other arm.

To save money and simplify your life, purchase hosiery labeled as "seconds" from catalogues. Also, limit your color choices in opaque hose and leggings to black and barely black; limit your color choices in sheer hose to natural or skin-toned, taupe, barely black, and black.

For a pulled-together appearance, pair a black skirt or an entire outfit of black with barely black or solid black sheer hose or leggings. With all other skirts and dresses, or when in doubt, wear sheer, flesh-colored hose. Just remember to get rid of leg hair since it can be seen through sheer hose.

Don't wear noticeable hose with sandals. Instead, if you like a smooth look to your feet and legs, try flesh-colored sandalfoot hose.

When you have on pants or a skirt with any type of shoe other than a sandal, you should also be wearing hose or at least opaque or patterned knee-high socks.

For dressier occasions, choose hose that is sheer and plain or has a little shimmer. With a simple dress, consider the allure of lace stockings.

Here's a strategy to use for your snagged hose. As you no doubt know, it's so irritating to put on a pair of pantyhose, discover a run, and be forced to start over with a new pair. To avoid repeating this scene, whenever you discover a run, seal the run off with clear nail polish and clip the inside label with scissors so you'll know to wear those hose only with full-length pants.

Socks are made in a variety of colors and styles. Too bad that they're appropriate only for casual occasions. Still, it's fun to have lots of eye-catching socks to wear with your loafers and boots, and even with your sandals.

Now that you know what to put on your feet, turn to the next chapter for the ways to add more pizzazz with your accessories.

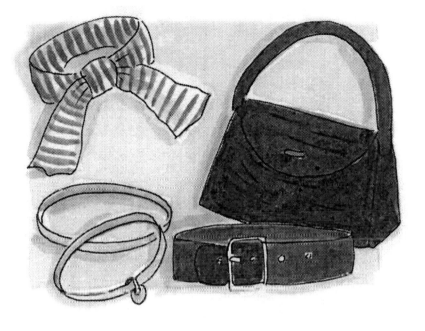

9

Make a statement with handbags, belts, scarves, and jewelry

Nothing says glamour and sophistication like showstopper handbags, belts, scarves, and jewelry. Because those accessories can be expensive, it's fortunate that you need only a few basic, classic pieces in your wardrobe. Here's another instance where you can concentrate on quality, rather than quantity.

The following is a summary of your "must-have" accessories.

Three handbags and a tote

Buy the very best handbags you can afford. Have three, all in black: one for fall and winter, one for spring and summer, and one for dressy occasions.

Your fall and winter handbag should be in textured black leather that will not show scratches and will last for years. In spring and summer, you'll want a black fabric handbag that can be machine- or hand-washed.

For dressy occasions, nothing is better than a black beaded handbag or a small purse in silver or gold metallic, just big enough to hold your wallet.

Don't overload your handbag. Periodically go through and pitch all unnecessary items. With your everyday handbag, try to confine yourself to carrying a small wallet, a day-timer or calendar book with a pen and pocket for business cards, a small cosmetic bag, a pocket-size packet of Kleenex, and an eyeglass case with a fabric eyeglass cleaner. If you carry a cell phone, choose a handbag with an inside pocket.

Before purchasing a handbag, test out its capacity to hold the items you typically carry. Here's how.

Transfer everything from your current handbag to

the one under consideration. Now, check to see if your prospective purchase has retained its original shape with no unsightly bulges. Walk around the store to see how it feels and glance at yourself in a full-length mirror to determine if it is the right size for your height and flatters the shape of your body.

If you decide against the purchase, be sure to return all your personal items to your own handbag. Once I forgot to do so, and had a few embarrassing moments, as I started to leave the store, oblivious to the fact that the un-paid-for handbag with all my personal paraphernalia was still on my shoulder. Suddenly, I heard the loud shrill of an alarm and saw clerks rushing around to locate the culprit. After I confessed that I was the one, they accepted my explanation and didn't call the cops. Even though I appreciated their understanding, I waited about a month before returning to that store.

To spruce up an outfit, consider a handbag in a color that either blends with or complements the color of your shoes. For example, with your black shoes, try a plain taupe handbag or a black handbag trimmed or embroidered in a contrasting color.

You can always use a tote bag, if only to carry an umbrella, newspaper, or magazine. As recommended in

Chapter 3, if a tote bag is part of your work or business-like ensemble, do not carry a handbag at the same time. Instead, carry your personal items in a small purse or separate zippered bag that can be placed inside the larger tote.

Be sure to weatherproof your handbags and tote with a protective spray designed for that purpose. Always read the label of the spray can to check whether the spray is recommended for use with the material or fabric of your handbag or tote.

Belts

You need only three basic, good quality, leather belts in your wardrobe: two in black and one in brown.

To know what length of belt to buy, keep in mind that a belt should be buckled on the third notch.

When you shop for a belt of a certain width to wear with a pant or skirt that has belt loops, take a piece of cardboard with you that is cut to the exact width needed. As a versatile option, consider a thin belt that can be worn inside belt loops of different widths.

To show off a unique belt, don't make the mistake of wearing it with lots of jewelry. Instead, let your belt be the focus of attention.

Scarves

Talk about pizzazz! Nothing adds punch to an outfit like a scarf. With the use of a scarf, you can take a dressy outfit down a notch or turn an ordinary outfit into a fashion statement.

To avoid a washed-out look when your outfit is all black, brown, or charcoal gray, add a scarf in one of your best colors or choose a color everyone can wear; that is, periwinkle blue, turquoise, coral, or soft white. Or, try a pink scarf to magically give your face a rosy, healthy glow.

Treat yourself to an expensive scarf every so often. You deserve it, and it's a purchase that will literally last a lifetime. I'm wearing scarves I inherited some twenty years ago from my aunt.

Have fun trying out different, innovative ways to wear your scarves. Here are a few suggestions:

- *In a slip knot:* double an oblong scarf to form a loop with two loose ends, wrap the scarf around your neck, and pull the two loose ends through the loop.

- *To fill in your neckline:* fold a 36" square scarf into a three inch rectangle and tie it around your neck by folding one end over the other.

- *As an accent:* place an oblong scarf under the lapels of or inside your jacket with the ends knotted or hanging freely.

- *As a kerchief:* fold a 36" square scarf across the diagonal into a triangle to wear on your head and tied under your chin.

- *As a cowboy tie:* fold a 36" square scarf into a triangle and tie around your neck in a loose, square knot.

To learn about all the different ways to wear scarves, consult one of the many available books that provide step-by step instructions. A word of caution: because styles change for scarves just as they do for most clothing, check to see how fashion designers are currently using scarves in their clothing lines.

Jewelry

Better to collect jewelry to wear than to collect figurines that just sit in a hutch or bookcase. A friend of mine recently said she was no longer spending money on anything for her house; that is, no more tables, chairs, bookcases, sofas, or knick-knacks for her. She has decided to invest instead in the clothes on her back and the trinkets on her arms.

An outfit of all one color is the best way to showcase your jewelry. Picture your favorite necklace and pendant with a simple black dress.

You may want a signature piece of jewelry or a collection of similar items you're known for wearing, such as animal images.

Be sure the size of your jewelry matches your frame. If you are a large-boned person, small or petite jewelry will be lost on you. If you are a small-boned person, large jewelry will overwhelm you. Check yourself out in a full-length mirror to make sure the size of the jewelry is right for you.

Before you buy more jewelry, know whether the undertone of your skin is cool (blue-based) or warm (yellow-based). If you're uncertain or it's been some time since your skin tone was analyzed, consult an expert in face products at a well-known store in your area or an expert who identifies colors by seasons or another similar system.

As a general rule, if the undertone of your skin is cool or blue-based, you'll want to invest in sterling silver, white-gold, and platinum jewelry. To flatter a warm or yellow-based undertone, the better choice is yellow-gold, brass, copper, and vermeil jewelry.

A color analysis expert may also be able to tell you

which jewelry styles become you. For example, if you have a long neck and an oval-shaped face with a square jaw, you look wonderful in geometric shaped jewelry.

Earrings don't mix well with eyeglasses that you wear all the time. To avoid a cluttered appearance, nix those hoops and long earrings as they will distract from, rather than enhance, your face. Limit yourself to stud earrings and add glamour with other jewelry, such as a fabulous watch, layers of bangle bracelets, or a gorgeous ring.

With reading glasses, you might get by with simple earrings of no more than one inch in length. If your everyday eyeglasses are rimless, you may be able to wear long earrings with a plain outfit, but it's an iffy proposition.

When you look in a full-length mirror, and see nothing but glitter, you have loaded yourself down with too much jewelry. Start taking your jewelry off, piece by piece, until your look is simple and perfect.

Nametags belong on your upper right-hand side of your jacket, blazer, dress, or worn-alone top, such as blouse or tunic. When people greet you, they can look at both your face and nametag at the same time. Test this out with a friend.

None of your jewelry has to be the "real" thing.

Sterling silver and white-gold look almost identical, and silver jewelry is often layered with a non-tarnish or platinum finish. Vermeil is the look-alike for yellow-gold.

Cubic zirconia and other look-alike "diamond" earrings can easily pass for real diamond ones if their total weight is no more than one and a half carats.

Here is a list of the basic staples in jewelry:

- Three chain or rope necklaces in 16",18", and 20" inch lengths
- Three pendants
- Pearls in 18" length
- Three pins or brooches
- Watch
- Hammered bangle bracelet
- Simple link bracelet
- Look-alike or real diamond stud earrings
- Pearl stud earrings
- Ball stud earrings
- Three-quarter-to one-inch hoop earrings
- Simple ring and a semi-fancy ring

After you've decked yourself out with jewelry and are the envy of Ms. Got-Rocks, you'll want to take a well-deserved break. Just don't get too comfortable because your next step is to audit your present wardrobe, get rid of those items you no longer value, and organize what remains.

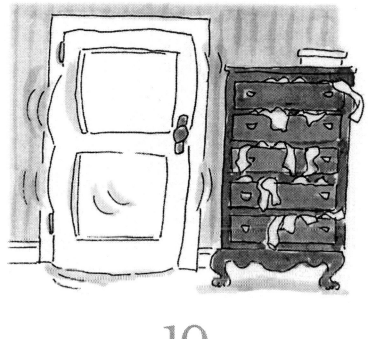

10

Audit and organize your current wardrobe

Now is the time to let go of those clothes and accessories you no longer wear or love. Vow to keep only what you value and know to be beautiful.

Cleaning out your closet

It's important to start fresh. Your task is to get rid of everything that doesn't fit, hasn't been worn in three years, and no longer serves your lifestyle needs.

As you go through the process of removing the excess from your drawers and closets, you can either make one big pile to deal with later or separate your discards into four piles designated for repair, consignment, charitable donation, and the trash.

The easiest way to start is to quickly go through and remove the clothes, shoes, gloves, handbags, lingerie, and robes that you haven't worn in the past three years. The only exceptions are jewelry, scarves, and dressy jackets, those classics pieces you love that will always be in style.

Wave goodbye to those items that were expensive, but for one reason or another, you never wore. Remember that almost everything you buy, such as a new car, decreases in value the minute you take possession. You might want to adopt a new attitude: all your new clothes and accessories lose their price tags the minute you bring them home. Whether they stay on a temporary or permanent basis depends on how useful they are to your present lifestyle.

Take a critical look at the remaining clothing and accessories. Try everything on in front of a mirror. Don't keep anything that is beyond repair, out of style, or unflattering, such as pants or jackets with pockets that don't lie flat.

Moreover, don't clutter your closet with clothes that are ripped, frayed, piled, tight, out of shape, too big, or which bulge in the wrong places or cling to your body as if you got dressed while taking a shower.

As mentioned in Chapter 2, be sure to toss all T-shirts that have juvenile or outlandish messages written on them and all clothing that looks like it belongs to your daughter, granddaughter, or the next door neighbor's teenage niece. We're talking short-shorts, mini and ruffled skirts, halter-tops, slip dresses, leather jeans, and anything with all-out cleavage. Also, dump the false eyelashes and purple lipstick.

Don't forget about the garments like transparent tops that make you uncomfortable just thinking about wearing them. And there are also those items you tired of and no longer want to keep, based on "GP" or general principle.

Unless you've already separated your discards into four piles, it's time to weed through your to-be-tossed pile. If you find some items you absolutely love that would be like new if fixed or tailored, put them in your repair pile. Examples are clothes with a missing button or jackets with sleeves to be shortened.

When you discover an item about which you are

sentimental, like your graduation dress from high school, take a picture of it for your scrapbook and, with a fond farewell, add the item to your consignment or donation pile.

The clothes and accessories that still have some life left in them for someone else's use, can be separated into two piles, one for consignment and the other for charitable donation. When you deliver those items to their respective places, be sure to get a dated and signed receipt that describes each item and specifies its value for consignment or tax purposes.

The remainder in your discard pile should be those items that are beyond repair and so worn that the only place they belong is in the trash.

Organizing what remains

Since you've gone this far, you might as well organize your closet. Here are some ideas.

Consider installing two rods, one on top of the other, to hang two tiers of clothes. Otherwise, I recommend that you just live with your closet as is. It's not all that difficult to convert any closet into a streamlined, organized delight.

First, take absolutely everything out of your closet. Before you shift through your clothes to see what to store in other places and what belongs in your regular closet, I recommend that you consider making a list of all the clothes you own. This list will come in handy when you create your future simple wardrobe.

Your next step is to decide where to store out-of-season clothes and dressy outfits worn only on special occasions. You could fold and store them for safe-keeping in boxes or on a shelf in your closet. Another option is to store them in a spare closet with mothballs or cedar cakes until time to transfer them back to your regular closet.

You're now ready to hang and organize this season's clothing in your closet. Separate your skirt suits into two pieces, skirt and jacket, and do the same with your pantsuits. Put like items together (pants, skirts, tops, and jackets) and organize them by color starting with black in the back and forwarding to white. To minimize wrinkling, don't squash your clothes together.

Treat your clothes to thin but sturdy velvet or suede hangers. Your pants will look their best when hung by their cuffs on clip hangers or hung over open-ended or four-tier hangers. Use belt rings for your belts and cup hooks, lined up in a row, for your necklaces.

Although I have read that knitted garments retain their shape best if kept in a drawer or on a shelf, I ignore such advice. I've found I don't wear my knits unless I can readily see them. My solution is to only hang those knits I'm currently wearing and store the out-of-season knits in drawers or on closet shelves.

If I find that one of my knits has "grown" while hanging, I transfer it from the hanger to a drawer or shelf. Whenever I decide to wear that knit, I allow extra time for steaming out any wrinkles.

You may be curious about whether, in fact, you wear all your clothes during a particular season. Here's how to find out.

After you've worn an item and re-hung it, return that hanger to the clothing rack in your closet. Re-hang that hanger in the opposite direction of the hangers with the yet-to-be worn clothes. At the end of the season, take a look at the hangers to discover which clothes have never made it out of the closet.

Until recently, I had forgotten all about my lovely scarves. I had made the mistake of neatly folding them in a drawer that I seldom opened. To correct the situation, I now display them in my closet on stackable clip hangers.

I have read that the average American woman has at least thirty pairs of shoes. Try to organize your shoes by color and store them in their original or plastic boxes, or on a shoe rack. Some women take Polaroid pictures of their shoes and tape the photos to the boxes. I just rely on the descriptions printed on the sides of the shoeboxes.

Keep your closet and drawers clear of clutter by keeping a box or assigning a certain space in your closet for items to be consigned or donated. If a garment needs repair, either mend it yourself or take it to a tailor or dressmaker. For anything that has seen its last day, trash it.

Other storage spaces

Separate your hose by color in individual open boxes in a chest or dresser drawer. I use lidless shoeboxes to organize my hose.

Full- and half-slips can be hung in your closet, or folded and placed on a shelf or in a drawer.

If you have limited space in your closet, you can fold sweaters and T-shirts, and store them on a shelf or in a drawer. The drawback is that it's difficult to remove an individual one from the stack. Some people solve this problem by rolling their T-shirts and sweaters like sausages.

Another idea is to use the linen closet for your T-shirts, sweaters, and handbags and store your linens in plastic or metal boxes under the bed.

Whew! I know cleaning out your closet and organizing what remains is not easy. I've been there, done that. Thank heavens, you'll never have to do that again. Since your new wardrobe is streamlined and simple, it will be a snap to keep your clothes organized.

Let's move on to the next chapter to find out how to identify those clothes that make up your own private and public dress codes or uniforms.

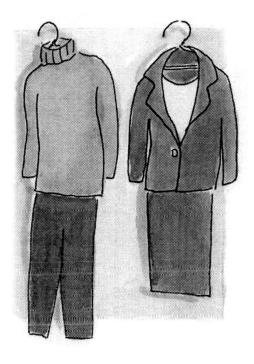

11

Discover your private and public dress codes

Your wardrobe is ideal when it combines what looks fantastic on you, what you love, and what you need.

The preceding ten chapters have been your guide to what looks great on you. Topics have included various types of clothes, the clothing details that enhance your body shape and make you look thinner and taller, the three colors for basics, your best colors for all other items, shoes for different occasions, and your accessories.

If you followed the instructions in the last chapter and audited and organized your closet, you know exactly what you have in your present wardrobe.

You're now about to discover how to identify what you love and what you presently wear or envision yourself wearing on different occasions; that is, your private and public dress codes or uniforms. You will find this information essential for creating your simple wardrobe that supplies all your clothing needs for a typical 14-day period.

The words "private dress code" and "private uniform" are used to describe those outfits that reflect your personal side, are physically and psychologically comfortable, or were purchased by you "just because." An example of your private dress code or uniform is the clothing you wear for relaxing or hanging out.

The words "public dress code" and "public uniform" are used to describe those outfits that fit the general public's expectations of what is suitable or appropriate in a particular situation or setting. An example of your public dress code or uniform might be the outfits you wear to work.

Private dress code or uniform

Even though you may indulge from time to time in the latest fashion items that everyone is talking about, you probably still find yourself wearing the same outfits every chance you get.

Those are the outfits that you depend on when you want to look and feel good, that you repeat in different fabrics and colors, and that you never grow tired of wearing.

Now is a good time to open your closet door and take a careful look at the clothes you grab over and over again. Those are the styles that reflect the real you; that is, your private dress code or your private uniform.

If you discover that all your clothes for easy dressing are of the same or similar style, you may question the wisdom of having such a limited selection. You might even conclude that, if you decided to wear the same or similar outfit most of the time, you would look boring to others, or even worse, to yourself.

Nonsense. When you look great, you feel great. Stick with the winners.

My favorites are my blue jeans, an olive jacket that goes with everything, a black knit pantsuit, and a three-piece, black, lightweight wool suit.

Take the time now to make a list in your notebook

of the different outfits that make up your private dress code.

Public dress code or uniform

How you dress affects the way you are perceived and treated. Regardless of whether you are employed, are the CEO of your own company, volunteer your services, or live the retired life, you need clothes that are suitable or appropriate for particular situations and occasions. Those clothes make up your public dress code or uniform.

First impressions make for lasting impressions. If you want people to pay attention to what you say and do, you must look the part you are playing. Study the public dress code of successful women who are in the same or a similar role as you.

Five different types of attire

Your dress codes or uniforms can be described or broken down into five, distinctly different types of attire, as listed below:

1. Formal business or professional attire

2. Casual business or professional attire

3. Informal, stylish, and chic attire

4. Dressy attire

5. Casual and relaxed attire

Each type of attire calls for specific clothes. When you create your perfect wardrobe, you may want to include outfits based on all five different categories of attire.

However, you may discover that there are one or more categories of attire for which you simply have no need. For example, you may be retired and no longer wear clothes designed for formal business or professional work. Or, you may not like to attend dressy functions.

Take the time now to read the questions set out below. Consider only those situations or occasions that are relevant to your lifestyle and ask yourself this question: what clothes do you or would you wear for:

1. Formal business or professional attire? In other words, what clothes do you or would you wear for work (employed or self-employed, full-time or part-time), business activities, and somber occasions such as baptisms, funerals, weddings, and graduation ceremonies?

2. Casual business or casual professional attire?
   In other words, what clothes do you or would
   you wear for relaxed business atmospheres,
   casual Fridays, creative work, volunteer
   activities, workshops, seminars, classes,
   and religious services?

3. Informal, stylish, and chic attire? In other words,
   what clothes do you or would you wear for a
   non-business luncheon, dinner, or party?

4. Your dressy attire? In other words, what clothes
   do you or would you wear for a cocktail party,
   banquet, or other dressy affair?

5. Casual and relaxed attire? In other words, what
   clothes do you or would you wear for relaxing,
   babysitting, hanging out, and chatting over
   coffee?

When you review your answers, you may find that
you now wear the same outfit or outfits for more than
one category of attire. For example, say you have, as
part of your wardrobe, an embroidered denim dress
with matching jacket and also a plain black pantsuit

that you love to combine with colorful T-shirts and sweaters. You now wear those two outfits as your casual business attire for your volunteer activities and also as your informal chic attire for luncheons. That would be good news.

However, when you think about all that you already own and the types of outfits you need for all your lifestyle activities, you might discover you have far too many clothes in one category and not enough in another. That would be bad news.

Don't panic. In the next chapters, you'll learn how to easily make use of all your clothes and fill in the gaps between your present and future wardrobes. For example, say you are semi-retired and no longer need a closet full of skirt suits for business. You could decide to keep the suit jackets to wear with pants, jeans, and khakis, and donate the suit skirts to a charity or sell them through a consignment shop.

Your final consideration is whether there are other situations or occasions that are not covered in the list of five types of attire. Take the time now to write in your notebook what you now wear or would like to wear in the future as attire for those specific situations or occasions.

Suggested outfits for special occasions

When you can't decide what to wear on special occasions, consider these ideas:

- *Class reunion:* jewel-tone dress or pantsuit in the latest style, fantastic looking shoes and handbag, and minimal jewelry (you don't want to look like you're trying too hard)

- *College graduation:* knee-length skirt suit that skims your body, classic jewelry, and low-heel pumps or flats if you will be on your feet most of the time

- *Milestone religious events such as a baptism, confirmation, or bar mitzvah:* skirt suit with a blouse in white or one of your best colors, or a shift-style dress with a print or patterned cropped jacket, and black mid-heel pumps

- *Lavish luncheon or afternoon party:* black dress with silk floral print jacket

- *Outdoor evening party:* khaki pants; tucked-in, white silk blouse; white jacket (try rolling the blouse sleeves over the jacket sleeves); pearls; beige belt; tan chunky low-heel pumps or sandals (no thin heels as you will be outdoors); and eye-catching print or flowered cloth shoulder-strap bag

- *Summer evening cocktail party:* black or white ankle-length silk pantsuit; jeweled blouse; long, dangling earrings; and metallic mid-heel pumps with straps

- *Holiday party:* velvet pants, silk blouse, embroidered vest, and patent leather mid-heel pumps

Your signature piece

As mentioned in Chapter 9, you may want to adopt a special piece of clothing or jewelry as your own signature piece. Whatever you choose should make you feel like a million bucks. Maybe it's a gold brooch or lovely earrings that your favorite relative left you in her will. Perhaps it's a jacket that goes with everything from your jeans to the finest silk pants and is always in style. Or, you might like to be known by a distinctive, stylish handbag such as the Kelly Bag, or sunglasses like the ones worn by Jackie Onassis.

Enough said. Take a deep breath because, armed with all the information you've gathered from the first eleven chapters, you are now ready to create your own perfect, personalized, simple wardrobe — on paper.

The ancestor of every action
is a thought.

Ralph Waldo Emerson

12

Create your perfect wardrobe

You'll know your wardrobe is perfect when it consists of only those clothes that you need, love, and look fabulous wearing. Here's how to create that ideal wardrobe.

Combining all information

First, take out your notebook and review your list of activities during a typical 14-day period. Study your notes about the different types of clothing. Pay particular attention to the details that flatter your body type and make you look thinner and taller, your best colors, the shoes you need, and the accessories to add a touch of magic to your outfits.

Then focus on the clothes that reflect your private and public dress codes. Also consider whether you intend to wear the same outfit more than once during a 14-day period or will want a different outfit for each day.

After reviewing this information about what looks good on you and what you like to wear, you are now ready to outline your perfect wardrobe — on paper.

Two hypothetical wardrobes

Skip over this next section if you think you will have no trouble figuring out exactly what you need and will want to wear during a typical 14-day period.

Otherwise, study the following two hypothetical wardrobes mentioned earlier in Chapter 2, one for Jane Doe and the one for Sally Smith, to help you understand how easy it is to analyze and resolve your clothing needs for a 14-day period. Details about the colors, styles, and different types of clothing are not included in these two illustrations, but should be included in your own individual, wardrobe plan.

For clarity, before the discussion of the wardrobe plans for Jane Doe and Sally Smith, the lists of their activities are repeated.

Jane Doe works full-time for five days a week for an accounting firm that expects their employees to dress in business attire Mondays through Thursdays and dress-down attire on casual Fridays. On Monday, Wednesday, and Thursday nights, she goes to a local health club after work for exercise and weight lifting, and on Tuesday and Friday nights, she relaxes with her family. On the weekend, she does household chores, hangs out with family and friends, and attends a jazz concert on one night and dines out the other night. Occasionally, she is invited to a dressy affair.

Jane's wardrobe plan: Jane writes down the number of times (days, nights, or occasions) during a 14-day period that she plans to wear a certain kind of attire. For example, she needs eight days of formal, business attire for Mondays through Thursdays and two days of casual, business attire for dress-down Fridays.

Although she plans to wear her outfits more than once during a two-week period, she makes sure she has a sufficient variety of clothes, so she doesn't get bored with her wardrobe.

Her written 14-day wardrobe plan looks like this:

- *6 Outfits of formal business attire for 8 days of work on Mondays through Thursdays:*
  3 Skirt suits
  3 Pantsuits
  8 Blouses of different styles

- *2 Outfits of casual business attire for 2 dress-down Fridays:*
  1 Additional pantsuit
  1 Trouser pant
  1 Sharkskin blazer
  2 T-shirts

- *4 Outfits of informal, stylish, and chic attire for attending jazz concerts/dining out on weekends:*
  2 Pantsuits
  2 Dresses

- *3 Outfits of casual and relaxed attire suitable for 6 workouts on Mondays, Wednesdays, and Thursdays:*
  2 Jogging/exercise suits
  1 Blue jeans
  2 Loose tops

- *7 Outfits of casual and relaxed attire for relaxing after work on Tuesdays and Fridays, and doing household chores and relaxing with friends and family on weekends:*
  1 Casual dress
  6 Blue jeans/khakis
  1 Jean jacket
  1 Herringbone jacket
  3 Sweaters
  3 Additional T-shirts

- *1 Outfit of dressy attire:*
  1 Silk chiffon dress with matching scarf

- *Shoes:*
  Mid-heel pumps
  Low-heel pumps
  Low-heel dressy pumps
  Loafers
  Walking shoes
  Short boots
  Sandals

- *Handbags and tote:*
  1 Shoulder-strap bag
  1 Tote
  1 Sequin purse

- *Other items:*
  Raincoat with zip-out lining
  2 Other coats/ponchos
  Jewelry staples
  3 Belts
  Scarves

Jane compares the above 14-day wardrobe plan with her present wardrobe. She puts a check mark next to the items she already owns and makes a tentative list for future purchases, describing each item by color, style, type, and any other relevant details.

The second hypothetical is for Sally Smith who is recently retired from a full-time job. During a 14-day period, she volunteers her time at a local hospital for six mornings (Mondays, Wednesdays, and Fridays), and baby-sits her grandchildren for four mornings (Tuesdays and Thursdays). Her other weekday activities during a two-week period include attending two continuing education classes held on Wednesday and Friday afternoons, lunching with friends two or three times, taking long walks, going to the library, and relaxing at home whenever she can.

Sally attends monthly meetings at the Humane Society where she serves as a member of the Board of Directors. Occasionally, she meets with her banker and stockbroker.

On weekends, Sally attends religious services, does housekeeping chores such as grocery shopping and cleaning house, dines out with a movie afterwards, and relaxes the rest of the time. Whenever she can, she attends music concerts and art exhibits. About every other month, she is invited to a formal dinner party.

Sally's wardrobe plan: Sally still owns a number of skirt suits she no longer needs or wears. She selects her two favorite ones for Humane Society meetings and personal business activities; with the rest of her skirt suits, she plans to donate the skirts to charity and keep the jackets to pair with pants, jeans, and khakis.

Sally's written 14-day wardrobe plan looks like this:

- *2 Outfits of formal business attire for meetings such as at the Humane Society, and with her banker and stockbroker:*
    2 Favorite skirt suits (previously worn for work)
    2 Blouses

- *8 Outfits of casual business attire for volunteer activities (6 mornings), classes (4 afternoons), and religious services (on weekends):*
    4 Pantsuits
    4 Extra pants
    3 Jackets (from former skirt suits)

    1 Blazer
    6 T-shirts
    6 Sweaters

- *6 Outfits of informal, stylish, and chic attire for 2 to 3 lunches, 2 nights of dining out, and 1 to 2 nights at music concerts/art exhibits:*
  - 3 Casual dresses
  - 3 Knit pantsuits
  - 3 Silk or cotton T-shirts

- *10 Outfits of casual and relaxed attire for different activities, such as babysitting (4 mornings); taking long walks, going to the library, and/or relaxing at home (6 or more afternoons); doing housekeeping chores (2 days); and casual evenings (10 or more nights):*
  - 10 Jeans/khakis
  - 10 T-shirts

- *1 Outfit of dressy attire for a formal dinner party:*
  - 1 Long knit dress

- *Shoes:*
  - Low-heel pumps
  - Mid-heel dress pumps
  - Loafers
  - Walking shoes
  - Tennis shoes

Sandals
Boots

- *Handbags and tote:*
    1 Tote
    3 Shoulder-strap bags
    1 Dressy purse

- *Other items:*
    Raincoat with zip-out lining
    3 Other coats
    Jewelry staples
    Novelty jewelry
    5 Belts
    Scarves

As Jane did, Sally now takes stock of her clothes and, on her written wardrobe plan, puts a check mark next to the items she already owns. She also makes a tentative list for future purchases, describing each item by color, style, type, and any other relevant details.

As stated before, the two hypothetical wardrobes are included to give you an idea of how to create a perfect wardrobe — on paper. In the next two chapters, you'll find out how to make your dream wardrobe a reality, bridge the gap between your present and future wardrobes, and make shopping both easy and fun.

Your perfect wardrobe on paper

On new pieces of paper, copy your 14-day list of activities. Follow the same steps as noted above under the two hypothetical plans. In other words, figure out how many days, nights, or occasions you will wear particular types of attire, such as for work or casual business activity. Leave plenty of blank space after each type or category of attire.

With all your notes available for reference, fill in the blank spaces with a description of the outfits you want to wear. Include the number, type, style, color, and any other details that are important to you.

Don't forget to consider whether you are happy with a minimum number of clothes (content to mix and match individual pieces) or want more variety and a different outfit for each and every activity. Your choice depends on your level of comfort. Just try not to go overboard with either too few or too many clothes. Remember your goal is a simple wardrobe that you can easily manage.

Congratulations. You have just created your perfect wardrobe — on paper.

Plus one

If you're like me and like a wide variety of clothes to wear, you'll want to make sure you have enough options in your wardrobe to keep you happy. An easy way to accomplish this is to add one outfit to each category of clothes on your list.

For example, in Sally's wardrobe, she plans to have two outfits for formal business attire. She takes a pen to her list, strikes through "2," and inserts the number "3." For the remaining categories, she continues to do the same.

I'm not suggesting that you necessarily follow the "plus one" method of calculating how many outfits you want. However, you know yourself and you must do whatever makes you comfortable and happy. After all is said and done, this is about your own personalized wardrobe.

Additional 14-day plans

As mentioned in Chapter 2, if your activities change radically during the year, you will need to make extra plans. For example, if you are a teacher and you teach for nine to ten months and are on summer break for two to three months, you need two different 14-day plans: one for work and one for the summer break. Also, if you live in a part of the country that has different seasons, you will need more than one 14-day plan. For example, you might have one 14-day plan for fall and winter, and a second 14-day plan for spring and summer. Or depending on the weather in your area, you might want to devise four 14-day plans: one for each season.

If you normally wear most of your outfits for three seasons, another option would be to have a 14-day plan for fall, winter, and spring, and a second 14-day plan devoted to summer.

One way to simplify your wardrobe is to have several outfits in year-round fabrics such as matte jersey, wool crepe, and gabardines in wool and rayon blends.

After you are finished with the written plans for your perfect wardrobe, you are ready to take the concrete steps outlined in the next two chapters to make your dream wardrobe a reality.

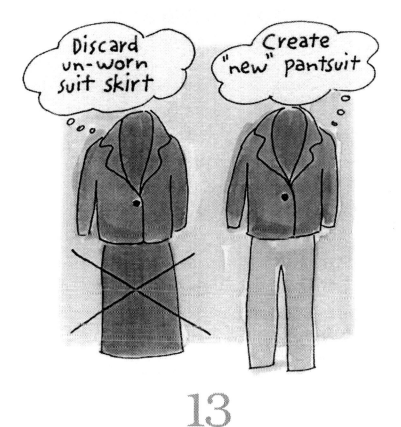

13

Make your dream wardrobe a reality

Integrating present with future

Take one last look at your existing wardrobe to make absolutely sure that what you now have is flattering and appropriate for your present lifestyle. You don't want to make the mistake of taking up space in your closet with clothes you never wear because they're inappropriate or fail to make you look your best.

As you go through this final audit, keep in mind two key ideas.

First, remember that you can pitch the skirts or pants of suits you no longer need and keep the jackets to pair with other pants, jeans, and khakis.

Second, decide if you can make some use of any skirts or pants that fit you perfectly and are almost like new, but unfortunately are not in a flattering color. Instead of pitching those skirts or pants, you could keep them to pair with a black or white jacket, and pull the whole outfit together with a scarf that has just a touch of the same color as the skirt or pant.

However, if all that seems like too much trouble, wave goodbye as you put those pants and skirts in the box or space in your closet designated for items you intend for future consignment or charitable donation.

After that last bit of auditing, you are ready to compare your present wardrobe with your written future wardrobe plans. If you haven't done so already, on your written plans, put a check mark next to those outfits you already own.

Filling in the blanks

It's so much easier to shop for clothes you need to make your wardrobe complete when you know what you're looking for. Prepare a written wish list for future purchases, describing them by color, style, type, and other relevant details. Also, be sure to read all about shopping in the next chapter.

Fit checkpoints

To look good, your clothes must fit! Make it a practice to check your clothes regularly to make sure none need alteration. It makes no sense to have a piece of clothing that is in one of your best colors, but, because it doesn't fit properly, just hangs in your closet, year after year.

Also, learn to be more discriminating in your choice of clothes. Limited options make for easier decisions. Promise yourself to spend money only on garments that do wonders for your body.

Here's a list of fit requirements for your present wardrobe and future purchases:

1. All pockets in skirts, pants, jackets, and dresses must lie flat.

2. No bulges, pulls, and smile lines are allowed in the hip, thigh, knee, crotch, and stomach areas; in other words, no bags, sags, or gags.

3. No puckers are permitted in the seams or hems of any garment.

4. The pleats of pants and skirts must lie flat.

5. A straight skirt or dress that hugs your body should fit perfectly, never too loose or too snug. It should fall straight from waist to hem without cupping or pulling in the front or back, and allow for walking by providing a slit or pleat in the skirt area.

6. Jackets should be capable of being buttoned or closed without pulling, and the back of your jacket should lie flat across your shoulders and hips.

7. Sweaters and blouses should never pull across or around your bust area; there should be no visible bulges.

8. Shoulders with set-in sleeves should fit at or be no more than one inch wider than the edge of your shoulder.

Taking care of your wardrobe

Make friends with a good dressmaker or tailor. Pay

particular attention to the length and hemline of your pants and skirts, and to the length of the sleeves of your jackets and coats. Remember, you can adjust the width of shoulders and, as needed, add, change, or remove shoulder pads.

As recommended in Chapter 5, when you have your skirts, pants, or dresses altered, take all the shoes with you that you will be wearing with those garments.

Your wardrobe represents an investment of your time and money. It's easy to wear the same jacket over and over again, and not realize that it needs cleaning Pick a number for the days you will wear an item before cleaning it; for instance, one to two days for washable clothes and three to five days for ones that must be dry-cleaned.

Make a special note of the garment care tag and follow it. If the tag says hand-wash, do not assume that the garment can be machine-washed on the delicate-cycle. Rather, place it in a mesh bag to protect it and keep it from spinning out of shape in the washing cycle.

If you are instructed to dry a garment on a hanger or a flat surface, you may be able to pre-dry it for one to two minutes in the dryer on the lowest heat cycle to smooth out any wrinkles made during the washing cycle. Thereafter, follow the exact instructions on the garment tag or label.

Your wardrobe savers are Static Guard, a crochet hook or other gadget to fix snags, tape rollers to remove lint, and a shoe kit consisting of brush, buffer, and neutral and black polish.

Since you've now completed your written wardrobe and know exactly what you need to buy to fill in the gaps, you are, no doubt, anxious and ready to head off to your favorite store or the mall. But before you do, read the next chapter to learn how to make wise purchases, how to avoid getting trapped by the sales rack, and how to buy trendy pieces on the cheap.

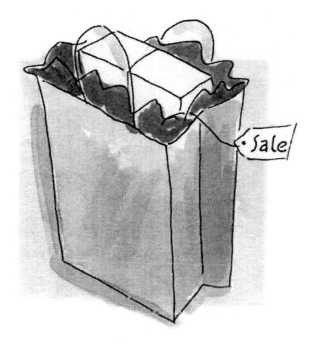

14

Shop smart and stay in style

Several years ago, my closest friend and her husband moved to Houston, Texas. When I went there for a visit, her husband would pick me up at the airport with this bit of news: "I contacted the major stores with your arrival date; they have been closed for the last two days to restock."

I can't help but smile just thinking about those days when I shopped till I dropped. I did learn a trick or two about shopping from those experiences, and I'm now going to pass my secrets on to you.

Details to consider

First of all, let's talk size. It is not in your best interest to allow yourself to be tyrannized by the size indicated on the tag of a garment for sale.

Having said that, I understand what a downer it is to go shopping, thinking you are one size, and then find you have to buy a size larger. Or you can try on a garment in a size smaller than the one you normally wear and become so enamored with what's happening that you immediately get out your charge card. Bad move! More likely than not, when you get your purchase home, you'll discover you don't look that great in it after all.

Accept the fact that if you are a size 12, you will be buying clothes than range from a size 10 to a size 14.

Different styles often require buying different sizes. For instance, when you shop for a pair of dress pants, if you plan to tuck-in your T-shirts and sweaters, you may have to go up a size; ditto for pencil skirts and straight-line pants.

Make a vow that, from now on, you will not allow the size of any garment to affect whether you buy it or not.

Instead, you will be taking a close look at its color and style and how you feel wearing it.

Insist on clothes that not only make you look fabulous, but are comfortable as well. The more at ease you feel in your outfits, the less time you'll spend thinking about your appearance.

Be sure to read the care label of the garment before you buy it. The major problem with owning clothes made of wool, silk, and some fabric blends is their upkeep. I hate dry-cleaning bills, along with the moth holes my clothes get when I try to wear them for that extra mile.

If the label of a garment reads "dry-clean" or "dry-clean only," think twice before you buy that item. Dry-cleaning is expensive! Chances are you can find a similar garment in a fabric that can be machine- or hand-washed, and dried in a clothes dryer, on a hanger, or on a flat surface.

Also, consider how much the particular fabric will wrinkle. If you love the look of linen, but hate how quickly it creases, only buy blouses and jackets in a washable linen blend.

Alone with the right tools

Shop alone, unless you have a friend who will give you

an honest opinion about what colors and styles look good on you.

To shop with ease, try "one-stop" shopping. When you find a store that has your kind of clothes, get to know the manager or one of the salesclerks. Tell that person what you like and ask to be contacted by phone or e-mail when something of your taste arrives or goes on sale.

Know why you are shopping and go armed with your color swatches and a list of clothes you need. When you just meander around, it is all too easy to make unwanted purchases.

You'll find it helpful to dress in a good-looking outfit when you shop; you will be treated well, while reminding yourself that you have plenty of great clothes, waiting at home for you to wear.

Your best tool in a store is a three-way mirror. I am always suspicious of a large store that doesn't have one. Don't they want me to see how I look in their clothes? Just in case, always carry a small mirror with you so you can see how you look from all angles.

Impulse shopping

Talk about dangerous! For your pocketbook's sake and a reality check, when you see an item you're interested in, ask yourself these questions.

First, and foremost, do I love it? Just sort of liking it isn't good enough.

Next, ask yourself, is it flattering? Look at yourself in a three-way mirror. Here's where a second opinion from a friend or a trusted salesclerk can be helpful.

Finally, ask yourself, where am I going to wear this? And when? Why do I think I need this now?

If you don't know the answers to those questions, you're about to purchase an item that will be worn, at best, only once or twice, and then banished to the back of the closet so you won't be reminded of your mistake. In other words, you're about to purchase clutter.

Still, regardless of how often we promise ourselves that we'll never again buy something just for the sake of buying something, we all have those days when, for one reason or another, we find ourselves in our favorite store or in the mall. Maybe we're there to see what's on sale, or just hanging out with a friend. Most of my mistakes have been at those times when I was out of sorts or depressed, and used shopping for therapy.

Try this strategy: when in doubt about a prospective purchase, don't buy it that day. Wait a week and see if you really, really want it. Should you decide to return to the store to buy it, only to find it's been sold to someone else, know that you were never meant to make that purchase.

In those situations, I try to console myself with the thought that there's no one piece of clothing that I absolutely have to have. Or is there? Hmmm.

Sales

Be careful when you go to sales, unless you're a seasoned shopper. Even though you know exactly what your wardrobe lacks, you may find it very hard to resist anything that is on the sale rack.

To avoid making a costly mistake, and before you make that purchase, ask yourself those questions listed in the preceding section on impulse shopping. Constantly remind yourself that a bargain's not a bargain unless you need it.

Wise investment pieces

Spend the most on those clothes that you will wear the most. In other words, the more costly the purchase, the more useful the item should be. For example, if you love wearing T-shirts with khakis or black pants, one way to vary your outfits is to own several different blazers. You could choose to buy inexpensive khakis, black pants, and T-shirts, and then splurge on stylish and classic blazers.

Here are the six qualities that make for an investment purchase:

1. You absolutely love it.

2. It is a classic.

3. With proper care, it will last several years.

4. You know exactly how it will mesh with the clothes and your lifestyle.

5. You look and feel fabulous in it.

6. It is on your list of clothes that make you feel and look like a million. Here's a list to get you started:

   • Simple, dark-colored, year-round, single-breasted blazer

   • Expensive, gorgeous scarf

   • Trenchcoat with button or zip-out lining

   • Anything in machine-washable suede

   • Black, year-round dress that is mid-calf or ankle-length and in a washable lightweight wool or fabric blend

   • Dressy cardigan sweater to wear instead of a jacket

- Off-white, black, or red cashmere turtleneck sweater that can be hand-washed
- Comfortable black leather pumps with one-inch heels
- Black leather shoulder-strap bag
- Bra that fits perfectly
- White- or yellow-gold bangle bracelet that is hammered and won't show scratches or dents
- White- or yellow-gold watch

Here's the list of items to skimp on:

- Jeans and khakis
- Straight skirts
- Extra skirts and extra pants
- Socks, pantyhose, and body shapers (buy "seconds" from a catalogue)
- Belts
- T-shirts, blouses, and sweaters in the latest fashion colors
- Casual summer dresses
- Hats
- Casual shoes such as sneakers and espadrilles

- Straw totes

- Anything that has to be dry-cleaned often, such as a white wool jacket.

- Anything that is of the moment, such as trendy jackets, wraps, and the latest jewelry.

Always in style

You'll want to know what's hot in today's fashion. To stay current, subscribe to at least one fashion magazine, such as *Vogue*, *Elle*, *In Style*, or *Harper's Bazaar*.

As mentioned in Chapters 3 and 7, you can easily and inexpensively update your wardrobe by adding a few inexpensive T-shirts, blouses, sweaters, shirt-jackets, or even costume jewelry in the colors of the moment (but only if those colors flatter you). Avoid wearing last year's colors, as they will make you look dated and stodgy.

To know what's on the cutting edge, watch for changes in the following:

- *Waistlines:* empire, at the natural waist, or below the waist?

- *Shoulder pads:* sharply defined or molded to the soft curves of a natural shoulder line, or none at all?

- *Pant legs:* straight or full?

- *Skirt hems:* at or below the knee, mid-calf, or longer?

What doesn't change is the necessity to be mindful of your hands, face, and hair. Don't skip the advice offered in the next chapter.

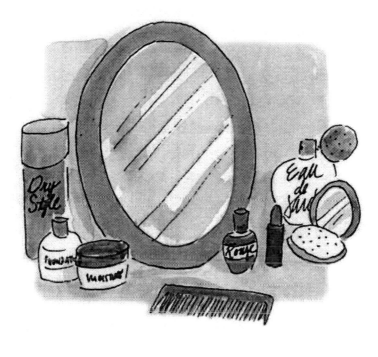

15

Don't forget your hands, face, and hair

As my Grandmother Marie Corn observed, "You can tell everything about a person, just by looking at their hands and feet."

Hands

Your hands reveal your age, and their condition says how much you care about your appearance.

Your nails must be manicured. As a minimum, treat yourself to a manicure every other week and a pedicure every other month.

Even if you have nails that are short, chipped, or ragged, I do not recommend that you apply false fingernails or even false tips. Your nails will look false and take center stage when you talk with others. The next time you are in the company of someone with fake nails, notice how they capture your attention. Instead, find a top-notch manicurist and get a weekly manicure until you can safely switch to every other week. Keep your nails short and protected with clear or light beige polish, and your hands soft with moisturizing lotion.

Skin care

The most important gift you can give your skin is a good moisturizer and sunscreen on your face during the day, and a rich cream on your face and body at night.

As you get older, age spots will start to appear. Fortunately, there are products on the market today that effectively fade those spots. I recommend applying a freckle remover at night to any part of your body where brown spots appear.

Makeup

Even though less is usually more when it comes to wearing makeup, only you can determine how much or how little makeup you need to look civilized. Here are a few suggestions.

Makeup should be soft, sheer, and flattering. Black liner is too overpowering for most faces, and heavy foundation and obvious color differences between your face and the rest of your body will add years to your appearance.

Pay attention to your eyebrows, as they frame your eyes. Go to a top-notch beauty salon and have a specialist tweeze them. A word of caution: when wax is applied under your eyebrows and above your upper lip, the skin can blister and burn. Some prescription medicine can cause your face to be sensitive. I know because I got burned once. I still have some faint scars.

It's important to use good brushes to apply your makeup. If you must, use eyeliner in a subtle shade of brown or taupe in the thinnest of lines on your upper eyelids next to your lashes. To avoid accentuating any bags under your eyes or giving your eyes a clown look, you might want to skip applying eyeliner to your lower eyelids.

As an alternative to eyeliner, try defining your upper

eyelids with powder eye shadow in a soft shade of brown.

Here's an easy routine to make sure you apply sunscreen. Right after you brush your teeth in the morning, immediately apply a moisturizer to your face and neck. Next, use sunscreen on any area exposed to the sun, such as your face, neck, and arms, but stay clear of the area around your eyes. For ease of application, you can buy moisturizer with sunscreen protection.

Your sunscreen (whether combined with moisturizer or not) should be hypoallergenic and PABA-free, with a SPF of 30 or more for UVA/UVB protection. Remember to check the expiration date on the bottle.

After a few minutes, you can brush your face with a mineral powder that is formulated to use alone. Or, pat on a little concealer or foundation to uneven or red areas and blend with your fingertip or Q-Tip, and then powder your face.

Next, smile and apply some pink or coral blush in either a powder or cream to the apple portions of your cheeks.

Fill in your eyebrows as needed with the same color they are naturally. Even if you don't use mascara, curl your eyelashes to give your eyes a more open look. If you want, finish with a coat of brown or black mascara.

Choose a matte color of lipstick that matches or is in a few shades lighter than your natural lips and, if you like, a lip liner that matches your lipstick. However, you may decide, particularly as you get older, that you don't want to unduly emphasize your lips and that you look best with just rosy lip gloss.

See if you can get by most days with only sunscreen, moisturizer, brow filler, blush, mascara, and colored lip-gloss.

Your last step is to spray your face with distilled water you keep in the refrigerator. Very refreshing. Then take one last look at your face. Smile to make sure you haven't filled any lines in your face with foundation or powder. If you have, blot your face and re-spray with water.

Don't forget to carry a small bottle of sunscreen in your makeup bag for applying throughout the day as needed.

For more information regarding creams and makeup to use, I suggest you consult a makeup expert in your area, and then follow-up with a second opinion.

Eyeglasses

If you wear prescription eyeglasses every day, they are

the single most important purchase you make, as your eyes are what people notice first when they look at your face.

At least every two years, you should familiarize yourself with the newest styles in frames to see if yours should be updated. It's amazing to me how many people fail to update their eyeglass frames or even get them adjusted for a proper fit.

Go to a store that has up-to-date, expensive eyeglasses. When I was in such a store this past fall, I had to wait until the clerk finished adjusting another customer's new eyeglasses. The clerk finally got to me with this explanation: "You'll have to excuse the wait, but, after all, when someone spends $1800 on eyeglasses, they expect to get my undivided attention." I'm not suggesting you go to that extreme, but don't choose one frame over another because it's $50 or even $100 cheaper. Remember, you will be wearing those glasses every day, and you deserve to look your best.

When you shop for new eyeglass frames, take one of your friends along for a second opinion and look at yourself in a full-length mirror to make sure the eyeglass frames are in proportion to your body.

You may want to have your eyes checked every year to see if there's any change in your prescription. If there is, you'll have an excuse to buy the latest eyeglasses. The lens should be non-glare, scratch resistant, and provide the latest eye protection.

If you have your vision corrected by LASIK or similar procedure, you may find that you need eyeglasses to read. Rather than hunt around for your reading glasses, while driving you and everyone around you nuts, hang them on a chain around your neck. Choose a chain in a style and color that looks good on you, or is in a neutral color, such as light tortoiseshell.

For sunglasses, here are some general guidelines. For a square-shaped face, consider an aviator style; for a round face, look for square frames; for a long face, the cat's eye is good; and, for a heart-shaped face, almost any shape is flattering.

Hair

Even though you're probably aware that you look disorganized with messy hair, you may not have the time to blow your hair dry and style it every day.

Hair should look understated. A cut that creates fullness and swings freely as you move your head is simply wonderful. Whatever style you choose, your hair should be simple to cut and easy to care for.

If your hair has some length, consider pulling your

hair back in a low ponytail as an alternative style. It can literally give your face a lift.

Talk to a good hairstylist about creating a style you can manage in 10 minutes or less, with minimum upkeep. If you don't have a regular hairstylist, look everywhere for someone with perfect hair, and then ask her for a reference.

As you get older, don't let your hair get longer than shoulder length. If you do, you'll look as if you're trying to look younger, when in fact, all you will have accomplished is to drag your face down and make yourself look older.

Hair of all the same color looks phony and is aging. At the same time, if you want to cover any gray hair, it's hard to find the right hair color to use. One option to make the gray hair less noticeable is to have your hair streaked about every other month with two different colors, one lighter than and one the same color as your natural hair.

To protect your hair and face when you spend a substantial amount of time in the sun, be sure to wear sunscreen and a hat.

Perfume and a last look

For a true luxury, when you're getting dressed, dust

your body with powder and spray yourself in fragrance. If you can smell your own perfume, you have too much on and need to sponge some off with a wet cloth.

Even if you're only headed for the grocery store, take a few minutes before you leave to look at yourself in a full-length mirror and make any necessary changes to your appearance. If you don't take the time to do so, you can bet money on running into someone you know. Why that happens, I have absolutely no idea. It just does.

To celebrate your new looks, consider taking a trip. You'll be sure to travel light if you pack using the wardrobe ideas outlined in the next chapter.

He who would travel happily
must travel light.

Antoine de Saint-Exupery

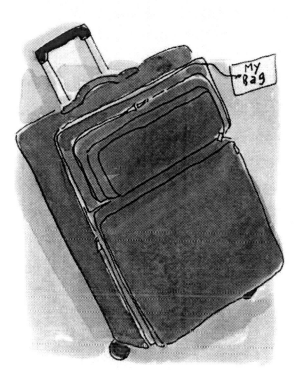

16

Travel light

Packing woes

You're all set to go. Or so you think. Suddenly, you remember you still have to pack. Feeling overwhelmed and clueless, you begin to ponder what you should take. Or what you should leave at home. Is less really more?

I heard about one woman who packed only her old "to-be-thrown-away" clothes for a trip. As she went about her travels, she discarded what she wore — item by item — and immediately bought something new as a replacement. When she got home, she had a suitcase full of brand-new clothes. Sounds tempting.

Because we have better things to do than fuss with our clothes when we are out of town, consider only easy-care, easy-to-wear garments with versatile styling that can take you through the day and into the night. Stick with fabrics that travel well and are wrinkle-resistant, such as polyesters, matte jerseys, and knits.

The easy way to travel

Here are six rules to abolish your clothing worries on any trip:

1. You must begin to pride yourself on how little you pack rather than how much. Try to start out with some room left over for items you will buy on your trip for yourself and others. To make life really simple, travel only with a small, carry-on piece of luggage on wheels and one large tote bag. Make it a rule that you never take more luggage than you can handle by yourself. That's the best way to banish forever the fear of lost luggage!

2. Start with a master checklist and have it available on your computer. When you are getting ready for a trip, print it out.

3. Try not to buy new clothes for your trip or take things that you don't wear at home. Pack only those clothes you like to wear and be sure that those clothes are comfortable. Make a space in your closet for the clothes you are taking on the trip. Start gathering other items, and put them on a table or shelf.

4. Take the time now to make a copy of your passport, driver's license, and credit cards, along with the number to call if you lose the cards. Put those copies with the receipt for your traveler's checks in the zipper part of your carry-on luggage.

5. Unless you're a rock star who is hounded daily by photographers, you don't need a new outfit for every day of travel. You can wear one pair of slacks or one skirt for three days and each of your T-shirts, pullover sweaters, and blouses for two days. For dressy occasions, you can add an

evening purse and either a silk blouse or matte jersey dress.

6. Build your travel wardrobe around basics in black, charcoal gray, or brown. I always choose black because I find it easiest to work with. Some women like to pack only knits. As a minimum, plan to take one pantsuit (or blazer and plain slacks) in your basic color and one pair of khaki pants or jeans (again, I recommend black). Add a third pair of slacks, Bermuda shorts, or a skirt. Take a raincoat with a zip-out lining. If it's cold where you're going, pack a warm scarf and gloves.

Your wardrobe for a 10-day trip

Your simple wardrobe for a 10-day trip now looks like this:

- 1 Pantsuit, or plain pant and blazer
- 2 Pants/slacks/khakis/jeans or 1 pant and 1 skirt
- 5 T-shirts/sweaters/blouses
- 3 Scarves and belt, if needed

- 1 Pair of sneakers or walking shoes

- 1 Pair of black low-heel shoes for dress

- 1 Pair of sandals or loafers (doubles as house slippers)

- Small evening purse and silk blouse or matte jersey dress

- Underwear, socks, and hose

- Raincoat (with zip-out lining)

- 2 Pajamas, or 2 nylon or polyester caftans

- Sunglasses

- Lint remover, shoe buff, pocket-size Kleenex tissue, and washcloth (if traveling outside the USA)

- Travel guide, maps, and small notebook; if needed, "hide-a-sock" or money belt for security

- Ticket, itinerary, and addresses for postcards

- *Small, tote umbrella

- *Small sewing kit and toilet wipes for travel outside USA

- *Medicine, written prescriptions, extra-strength aspirin or Tylenol, and toiletries, such as Q-Tips, cotton balls, eye drops, ear plugs, small emery board, and Band-Aids

- *Sunscreen, makeup, creams, moisturizer, and cologne to refresh (take "eau de samples"), all packed in Ziploc bags

- *Travel alarm, pocket calculator, electric appliances, and converter plugs (if needed)

- *Camera and film

  * Note: You may not be able to travel with some of those items. Be sure to check the current list of banned travel items and any other travel restrictions.

On the plane or train, plan to wear a pantsuit jacket or blazer, pants or jeans, sweater or T-shirt, and sneakers or walking shoes. Carry your raincoat. Label your suitcase and tote inside and out with your name and address, using, if you can, a business address to avoid making your home address available to would-be thieves.

Reading material and your everyday purse go in your tote bag, together with personal items. The tote bag will come in handy for shopping and, on your return trip, can be filled with goodies and gifts.

Call ahead to your hotel to find out if the following is included with your room: hairdryer, coffee maker, and sample toiletries.

Inspect the condition of your clothes a couple of days before your departure date. There is nothing worse (I've had this happen) than to get somewhere only to discover that your clothes don't fit the same way you remember, that your jacket or pant is missing a button, or that a zipper is shot. Wear a watch (if valuable, be sure it's insured) and plain rings. Add small nice earrings, like gold balls or pearls, but nothing dangling to get caught as you travel. You might want to buy yourself a few cheap necklaces or earrings for the trip, just for fun.

You are now ready to pack. I have rolled up my clothes, packed with tissue paper, put everything in plastic or cleaning bags, and, frankly, I get about the same results. So, I usually choose to pack with plastic sweater bags because they're easy.

Bon voyage!

You can't help getting older,
but you don't have to get old.

George Burns

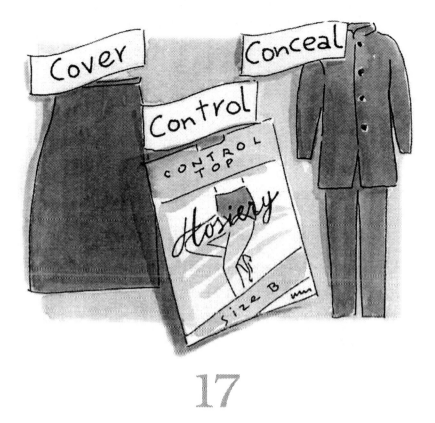

17

Gettin' old ain't for sissies

For many years I kept close ties with my aunt who lived in Kansas City. She was a spunky lady, hard to get along with, but always admired for her fabulous style, sense of humor, and zest for living.

She passed away when she was about 86 years old. It was hard to tell her actual age because she would never reveal the year she was born. I miss her.

My aunt had what some call attitude. The longer I

live, the more I think that it's all about attitude: an optimistic attitude about one's life and oneself.

My aunt gave me some tips to stay gorgeous as time goes by, and I incorporated them in earlier chapters. In the next section, I have repeated some of those tips and added a few of my own.

Tips

At some point you may find that all areas of your body, except for your mind (and memory), have increased in size. Do not be alarmed. Just adopt a new mantra: cover, control, and conceal. Here are some ways to maintain a youthful appearance:

- Be mindful at all times of your posture.

- Wear comfortable clothes so you can relax and enjoy yourself.

- Make sure your undergarments fit properly. A good bra can take years off your appearance.

- Cover your upper arms with short, long, or three-quarter length sleeves.

- Nix or fix any garment that bags, sags, or gags when you wear it.

- Before you leave the house, take a few minutes to look at yourself in a full-length mirror and make any necessary changes to your appearance.

- Include a belt with an outfit consisting of a tucked-in blouse or sweater, and a pant or skirt suit. When you have the suit jacket open with the front portion, but no more, of the belt showing, you give the impression that you have a small waist.

- Pair a flat-front pant or skirt that has a side-zipper and elastic in the back of the waist, with a mid-hip or longer top to cover the elastic waistband and zipper.

- Wear body shapers or control-top pantyhose with your pants and skirts to make sure your pants and skirts fit perfectly and fall straight down with no ripples whatsoever.

- Even though a particular brand of body shapers indicates you should wear a certain size for your height and weight, have a few extra on hand in the next largest size for those times, like the holidays, when you need some extra room.

- When you find that perfect pair of shoes, buy an extra pair to store away for future use.

- Your clothes must fit perfectly. No exceptions allowed. Even the most expensive garments can require some tailoring. Find a talented dressmaker or tailor to ensure you look your very best in all your clothes.

- Don't let your hair grow past your shoulders.
- To enhance, not overpower your face, wear stud, button, or small hoop earrings.

One last personal note: having determined that I need all the help I can get, I've made it my business to find out who is tops in their field or business. That is, I go to the best hairdresser, tailor, shoe repairer, and jeweler in town. I use two dry-cleaners, one for "good" clothes and another dry-cleaner for all other items. I also have made friends with knowledgeable salesclerks in my favorite stores, both in and out of town.

I strongly recommend that you find your own helpers. They can save you lots of money and time while providing you with professional services to keep you looking your best.

Congratulations

I'll close now by sending my congratulations to you for taking the time and effort to learn how to create, develop, and maintain your very own personalized, simple, fabulous wardrobe. Do yourself proud and wear it well!

Appendix 1: Bibliography / Recommended Reading

Arbetter, Lisa. *Secrets of Style: The Complete Guide to Dressing Your Best Every Day*. New York: In Style Books, 2003.

The following books that are part of the *Chic Simple Guides* created by Kim Johnson Gross and Jeff Stone.

Omelianuk, J. Scott. *Work Clothes*. New York: Knopf, 1996.

Urquhart, Rachel. *Women's Wardrobe*. New York: Knopf, 1995.

Worthington, Christa. *Clothes*. New York: Knopf, 1993.

Worthington, Christa. *Accessories*. New York: Knopf, 1996.

Eiseman, Leatrice. *Alive with Color: The Total Color System for Women & Men*. Washington, D.C.: Acropolis, 1983.

Feldon, Leah. *Does This Make Me Look Fat? The Definitive Rules for Dressing Thin for Every Height, Size, and Shape*. New York: Villard Books, 2000.

Feldon, Leah. *Dressing Rich: A Guide to Classic Chic for Women with More Taste than Money*. New York: Putnam, 1982.

Fischer-Mirkin, Toby. *Dress Code: Understanding the Hidden Meanings of Women's Clothes*. New York: Clarkson Potter, 1995.

Jackson, Carole. *Color Me Beautiful: Discover Your Natural Beauty Through the Colors That Make You Look Great & Feel Fabulous!* Washington, D.C.: Acropolis, 1984.

Larkey, Jan. *Flatter Your Figure.* New York: Prentice Hall Press, 1991.

Mathieson, Sherrie. *Forever Cool: How to Achieve Ageless, Youthful and Modern Personal Style.* Canada: Thompson Peak Publishing, 2006.

Molloy, John T. *The Woman's Dress for Success Book.* New York: Warner, 1977.

Molloy, John T. *New Women's Dress for Success.* New York: Warner, 1996.

Pooser, Doris. *Always in Style with Color Me Beautiful.* Washington, D.C.: Acropolis, 1985.

Rossbach, Sarah and Lin Yun. *Living Color: Master Lin Yun's Guide to Feng Shui and the Art of Color.* New York: Kodansha, 1994.

Sommers, Susan. *French Chic: How to Dress Like a Frenchwoman.* New York: Villard Books, 1988.

Woodall, Trinny and Susannah Constantine. *What Not to Wear.* New York: Riverhead Books, 2002.

Appendix 2: Web Sites

While there are many web sites for shopping, I have personally used and recommend the following:

www.drapers.com

www.easyspirit.com

www.eileenfisher.com

www.hsn.com

www.huffordsjewelry.com

www.jjill.com

www.landsend.com

www.llbean.com

www.neimanmarcus.com

www.norstrom.com

www.qvc.com

www.togshop.com

Sources for quotes

Page 6: Coco Chanel
www.womenshistory.about.com/

Page 30: Henry David Thoreau
www.quotationspage.com/

Page 38: Gilda Radner
www.quotationspage.com/

Page 54: Geoffrey Beene
www.brainyquote.com/

Page 64: Michel de Montaigne
www.quotationspage.com/

Page 76: Henry David Thoreau
www.quotationspage.com/

Page 92: Coco Chanel
www.womenshistory.about.com/

Page 130: Ralph Waldo Emerson
www.quotationspage.com/

Page 168: Antoine de Saint-Exupery
www.quotationspage.com/

Page 176: George Burns
www.quotationspage.com/

Page 187: Coco Chanel
www.womenshistory.about.com/

Index

I don't understand how a woman can leave the house without fixing herself up a little – if only out of politeness. And then, you never know, maybe that's the day she has a date with destiny. And it's best to be as pretty as possible for destiny.

Coco Chanel

Printed in the United States
106261LV00001B/4-153/A